A Case-Based Approach to State Hospital Psychiatry

A Case-Based Approach to State Hospital Psychiatry

MARTHA L. CROWNER, MD

OXFORD
UNIVERSITY PRESS

OXFORD
UNIVERSITY PRESS

Oxford University Press is a department of the University of Oxford.
It furthers the University's objective of excellence in research, scholarship,
and education by publishing worldwide. Oxford is a registered trade mark of
Oxford University Press in the UK and in certain other countries.

Published in the United States of America by Oxford University Press
546 Fifth Avenue, New York, NY 10036, United States of America.

CIP data is on file at the Library of Congress

ISBN 978–0–19–780058–4

DOI: 10.1093/med/9780197800584.001.0001

The manufacturer's authorized representative in the EU for product safety is
Oxford University Press España S.A. of Parque Empresarial San Fernando de Henares,
Avenida de Castilla, 2 – 28830 Madrid (www.oup.es/en or product.safety@oup.com).
OUP España S.A. also acts as importer into Spain of products made by the manufacturer.

CONTENTS

PREFACE

AIMS AND OVERVIEW

Many trainees and private-practice psychiatrists are strangers to modern state psychiatric hospitals. They may view them as vestiges of the past, offering only custodial care. This book presents what they can be: hospitals that serve seriously mentally ill people with effective treatment and careful discharge planning, hospitals where clinicians can find work hopeful and gratifying. This book also aims to honor the dedicated public service of state hospital employees and the struggles of patients under their care.

Compared to the more familiar community hospital inpatient units, state hospitals have a longer length of stay and serve a different, especially challenging population. Their patients are more likely to be seriously and chronically mentally ill and treatment-refractory. They often have serious medical problems and a history of involvement in the criminal justice system and of violent behavior. Some are patients who could not be safely discharged from community hospitals.

However, with a longer length of stay, public hospitals can accomplish what emergency rooms and short-term hospitalizations cannot. They can engage patients in treatment, identify and address what might contribute to poor treatment response, manage complicated medical and nursing problems, and contain and supervise dangerous individuals long enough for them to respond to treatment. With time, state hospitals can make discharge plans that give patients a chance to succeed outside of hospitals and jails.

This book is composed of summaries of clinically useful information, presented as discussions and shorter notes, interspersed with cases of state hospital patients. Cases are grounded in clinical experience but the patients are fictional. It also includes a few comments, which are the author's personal opinions. Some discussions and notes explain court cases and mental health laws and how they set the parameters of psychiatric practice. Most discussions are thorough, but not exhaustive, summaries of the scientific literature. These are written to be comprehensible and clear. They have a historical orientation and favor studies conducted in state hospitals.

Individual cases introduce a topic that nearby notes and discussions explore. All cases represent how severe psychiatric illnesses present and what to expect with long-term inpatient treatment. They illustrate how patients and their families contend with mental illness and the losses and disappointments it brings. Some show how public psychiatric care can be successful, and others show how it can fail.

SCOPE

For context and orientation the book starts with an overview of the history and recent functioning of state hospitals. The bulk of the book is composed of two groups of chapters, one on treatment and one on discharge.

Most cases describe individuals with difficult-to-treat schizophrenia or affective disorders. Discussions explore possible contributors to treatment refractoriness and means to address them. One is nonadherence. Due to the risk of nonadherence, long-acting injectables show superiority in preventing relapse. Persistent refusal can be addressed with medication over objection, but, to protect patients' rights, laws constrain its use.

Many patients who faithfully accept antipsychotic drugs have an inadequate short-term symptomatic response and fail to attain longer-term remission. They may be good candidates for clozapine. Clozapine offers hope not only for patients with treatment-refractory schizophrenia, but also for patients with schizophrenia who are at risk for violence or suicide, patients with polydipsia, and those with severe affective disorders.

Poor treatment response may be related to diagnostic inaccuracy. The book reviews the differential diagnosis of patients presenting with psychosis and considers how to understand the relationship between childhood abuse and adult psychiatric disorders. Self-reported childhood maltreatment is common in patients in public psychiatric care.

Discharge planning means finding a fit between an individual's needs and risks and available housing and services in the community. Patients can be discharged to family, but many lack family or need the supervision of supportive housing. Discussions describe types of housing and housing programs.

Discharge planning requires risk assessment and management. To aid in risk assessment the book includes a review of risk factors for violence. Risk management means providing adequate supervision. It sometimes entails leverage, which can be in the form of court-ordered community treatment, an alternative to incarceration program, or specialty parole or probation.

INTENDED AUDIENCE AND SUGGESTED USES WITH TRAINEES

The book's primary intended audience is students and trainees in psychiatry and other mental health fields as well as practicing clinicians. It should also be informative to family members or to anyone who cares for or has some responsibility for seriously mental ill adults. With trainees it can be used to learn about the treatment of serious mental illness, discharge planning, how to interpret the scientific literature, and simple statistics. Cases provide an anchor for clinical knowledge and an entry point for group conversations and presentations of similar cases. Together, the discussions are an easily accessible collection of synthesized information most relevant to working with state hospital and other seriously mentally ill patients.

GENERALIZABILITY

The patients in this casebook are not representative of all seriously mentally ill adults. Public hospitals have come to specialize in the care of involuntary and forensic patients. Forensic patients are by definition involved with the criminal justice system. Involuntary patients are ill to the degree that they are dangerous to others or themselves or unable to care for themselves. In general, public hospitals treat the most severely ill of a much larger group of people with serious psychiatric illness. Such patients exist in other countries and in all states in the United States.

The scientific literature summarized in this book applies across borders. The legal framework described varies somewhat, but not dramatically, across US states, and may vary in other countries.

Other contents of this book are less generalizable. The programs and procedures of the hospitals described in cases are individual and may not be similar in other locations or in other times. As well, community services described may not be available in other locations or in other times.

1

STATE HOSPITALS PAST AND PRESENT

This chapter reviews the history of public hospitals for psychiatric treatment in the United States and summarizes historical memoirs of former patients in these institutions. It details how this system for long-term psychiatric care and treatment began with a limited mission, expanded to attempt to meet a much broader mission, and then shrunk dramatically. The chapter ends with a brief overview of the current system.

1.1 COLONIAL TIMES TO 1890

1.1.1 History from 1773 to 1890

In colonial times, families were expected to care for dependent relatives, be they orphaned, physically handicapped, incapacitated and elderly, or severely mentally ill. When families could not do so, laws dictated that the community take responsibility. Arrangements for the care of mentally disabled persons took various forms; for example, local communities would pay for boarding with private citizens. Some mentally ill people were confined, but, in general, they were not confined involuntarily unless they were considered dangerous (Grob, 1994).

The first US hospital solely for the mentally ill, called the Public Hospital for Persons of Insane and Disordered Minds, admitted its first patient in 1773, in Williamsburg, Virginia. Its mandate was to provide short-term care in a crisis. It explicitly excluded troublesome alcoholics, the indigent, and chronically mentally disturbed people who were considered harmless (Zwelling, 1985).

Enthusiasm for *moral treatment*, purportedly capable of amelioration and even cure of mental illness, was characteristic of the early 1800s, a time of activism and optimism (Gollaher, 1995). "Moral treatment" is an Anglicized version of the original French *traitement moral*, coined by French innovator Philippe Pinel. In this context, the French *moral* did not mean virtuous, but mental or psychological. The approach called for confinement inside asylums with minimal use of restraints, where the asylum itself was the mainstay of treatment.

By 1830, US asylums in all parts of the country were insufficient to meet the enormous unmet need. In 1833, an asylum opened in Worcester, Massachusetts, providing moral and medical treatment. According to its first superintendent, between 1833 and 1845 at least 82% of its patients who had been ill a year or less recovered. With such encouraging reports of success, the Worcester asylum became a model for others (Grob, 1994).

In 1843, Dorothea Dix published her *Memorial to the Legislature of Massachusetts* (1904), in which she documented the horrendous care of mentally ill Massachusetts residents in jails and almshouses or boarded with private citizens. With her *Memorial* she argued that the mentally ill were helpless and suffering fellow humans whose care was a state obligation. Dix successfully lobbied members of the Massachusetts legislature to pass a bill funding an expansion of the Worcester asylum, which the governor signed. After her success in Massachusetts, Dix broadened her lobbying campaign. She asserted that because asylum treatment cured and allowed patients to return home, it saved money. In addition, she used examples of terrible crimes committed by insane persons to contend that asylums would prevent violence by containment (Gollaher, 1995). Over the course of 30 years she convinced legislatures in 18 states to found 32 asylums that would employ moral treatment (Sharfstein, 2000). These state institutions were the beginnings of the US public mental hospital system.

Usually, families made the painful decision to commit mentally ill relatives to state asylums. Their decision came only when there was no alternative: in the case of violence or threats of violence, suicidal behavior, severe depression or agitation, or when a caregiver died. Superintendents modeled their practice in public asylums on moral treatment. In addition to kind, individualized care in small institutions, patients were offered exercise, amusements and games, active employment in the hospital and on its grounds, and a daily routine. Superintendents prescribed drugs including morphine and opium, cathartics and tonics, but treatment also relied on individual counseling.

While states paid for building asylums, local governments or counties paid for the care and treatment of their indigent citizens residing in them. Counties saved money by exerting pressure to discharge and minimize the number of admissions. By law, only dangerously mentally ill people had to be admitted; others could be placed as county officials decided, often in cheaper almshouses.

Often, superintendents themselves had little authority to limit admissions. Most facilities suffered from insufficient funds because how much counties paid was often below costs incurred and slow in arriving. With time asylum populations grew and treatment quality suffered. Superintendents and their assistants had little time to meet with patients and became managers instead of therapists, concerned with staffing and maintaining large institutions (Grob, 1994).

By the 1860s, it became clear that asylum treatment, as it had evolved, was not as effective as advocates expected. Many people with severe neuropsychiatric illness could not be cured. In 1877, Pliny Earle, a leader among superintendents, wrote that members of his profession had systematically exaggerated recovery rates. Late in her career, even Dorothea Dix changed her views and advocated for clean, decent, and respectful custodial care, whether or not asylum's residents could be cured (Gollaher, 1995).

1.1.2 Anna Agnew's reminiscences

Memoirs are prone to bias, but they describe some patients' experiences of care and treatment. In *From Under the Cloud; or, Personal Reminiscences of Insanity*, Anna Agnew (2016) recounted her 1878 to 1883 stay at the Indiana Hospital for the Insane. When severely depressed and psychotic, she gave her young son a large dose of laudanum to spare him a later life of insanity. Her husband initiated commitment proceedings, and a physician certified that she was insane.

On arrival, she was grateful and relieved to be in a place where others acknowledged she was insane. The Indiana Hospital provided for Agnew's basic needs and offered a regular routine, employment, fresh air, and some diversions. She wrote that some attendants and physicians were kind and respectful, while others were abusive and contemptuous.

Because she made an attempt to hang herself in the Hospital, a physician ordered attendants to secure her arms in restraints when she retired for the night. When she refused to eat because her food "would become alive, creeping, squirming vermin," she was force fed (Agnew, 2016, p. 68). Physicians made rounds, spoke with her, and managed her nightly dosing of chloral hydrate (a sedative).

Anna Agnew left Indiana Hospital for the Insane to live with her sister for 10 years, until 1894, when she suffered a relapse and was admitted to a state hospital in Pennsylvania. There she stayed for 23 years until her death at age 80 (King, 2002).

1.1.3 Clifford Beers's memoir

In *Clifford Beers: A Mind that Found Itself* (2009), Beers chronicled his stay in a state asylum in Connecticut. He was first admitted to a private hospital in 1900, at the initiation of his family after he jumped out a second story window in a suicide attempt. In 1902, after he became manic, a judge ordered his transfer to a state facility. He commented, "private institutions are prone to shift their troublesome cases to state institutions" (Beers, 2009, p. 74). Clifford Beers was more critical than Agnew, though he had praise for some attendants and some doctors. His book contains a series of accounts of his struggles with hospital staff when he was combative, destructive, and "noisy." He admitted that, in his manic frenzy, he punched attendants and an assistant physician.

1.2 HISTORY FROM 1890 TO 1955

1.2.1 Unsustainable growth

A change in which particular government entity paid for care motivated counties to send needy citizens to asylums instead of almshouses. The change began with the New York State Care Act of 1890, which shifted the cost of state hospital care from New York counties to New York state. Most other states followed suit. County officials moved large numbers of older people out of almshouses, which county governments paid for, and into asylums, which state governments paid for (Grob, 1994).

Long-term psychiatric hospitals came to serve the functions of present-day nursing homes and assisted living facilities, institutions that only became common after World War II (Grob, 1980). Thirty to forty percent of all first admissions to state psychiatric hospitals in the 1920s, 1930s, and 1940s had a neurologic diagnosis that included Alzheimer's disease, arteriosclerosis, Huntington's disease, a brain tumor, or paretic neurosyphilis (Grob, 1994). Many newly admitted patients were elderly; some of these had dementia, but some did not. In 1930, of patients admitted to New York state psychiatric hospitals, 40% were older than 60, while 13.2% of the state's population was older than 60 (Grob, 1992).

Between 1911 and 1920, about 20% of all first admissions to New York state hospitals, the largest system in the country, were afflicted with paretic neurosyphilis, also called *general paresis* (Grob, 1994), a late manifestation of syphilis that causes progressive cognitive and physical deterioration. In the early 1900s, it required years of intensive nursing care before it uniformly ended in death. The incidence of neurosyphilis declined rapidly in the 1950s (Adams et al., 1997).

As long-stay patients comprised a growing proportion of hospital populations, the predominant function of state hospitals became long-term custodial care, more so than in the 1860s, when Dorothea Dix quit promoting them as instruments of cure. This occurred even though many, if not most, state hospital patients were treated and discharged. Elderly patients with dementia were rarely discharged and usually died in state hospitals (Kramer et al., 1955). Patients with schizophrenia were often admitted as physically healthy young adults and grew middle-aged or old in hospitals. In the early 1960s, the median stay for patients with schizophrenia in 13 states was almost 13 years (Grob, 1994).

During the Great Depression underfunding contributed to the deterioration of hospital physical plants, long waiting lists, and more crowding. As large numbers of American workers were pulled into the World War II effort, state hospital staffing was neglected. In 1943, in New York state, 31% of medical positions and 32% of ward staff positions were not filled (Grob, 1994).

At its peak, in 1955, the total population of all US public psychiatric hospitals was almost 559,000 (Manderscheid et al., 2009). The state hospital system had become unsustainable. Care for the mentally ill created an enormous burden on state governments. For example, in New York, it accounted for 38% of the State Purposes budget. In some states, hospitals were overcrowded by as much as 50%.

Even with their large capacities, state hospitals did not have enough beds to accommodate all the individuals who needed their services (Gorman, 1956).

1.2.2 *The Snake Pit*

In 1946, Mary Jane Ward published *The Snake Pit*. Ostensibly a novel narrated by V. Cunningham, it was based on Ward's own illness, identified as a "breakdown," and on her care and treatment at Rockland State Hospital in New York state. The book is notable for detailed descriptions of daily living conditions in that hospital.

The hospital cared for her basic needs, but minimally, because crowding and scarcity pervaded every aspect of patient life. "There wasn't enough of anything but patients," Ward wrote (1946, p. 253). "Not enough doctors, not enough nurses, not enough toilet paper, not enough food, not enough covers for cold nights." Lacking chairs for every woman in the dayroom, some sat or lay on the floor.

At times patients sat idle on the wards looking at nothing; at other times the hospital provided activities. The narrator attended a dance for both male and female patients with live music. She was also assigned jobs in the hospital.

The course of her treatment, primarily with electroconvulsive therapy (ECT), was rocky. At times she was paranoid, once she bit a psychiatrist, at one point she refused to eat and was force fed. The wards were run by powerful nurses, while doctors made irregular, brief appearances. The nurses' main goal was to keep patients quiet. To that end, some were put in straightjackets, some were restrained in tubs filled with water, and some were required to take paraldehyde, a sedative, at night. V. Cunningham—and Mary Jane Ward—finally recovered.

1.2.3 Rockland State Hospital 1931–1942

A review of administrative records from its opening in 1931 to 1941 (Keefe-Cooperman et al., 2024) provides a different view of Rockland State Hospital. In 1940, inpatients numbered 6,597. Most (54%) were diagnosed with *dementia praecox*, now called schizophrenia. Patients with neurologic illness comprised 22% of the population. Less-common diagnoses were bipolar disorder at 5%; alcohol abuse, 3.4%; mental deficiency, 2.1%; and primary behavioral disorder, 1.9%.

The hospital grounds covered 613 acres and included a power plant, bakery, laundry, and firehouse. Staff members, the majority of them attendants, usually lived on grounds. Less-impaired patients worked the on-site farm or manufactured mattresses, visited the soda fountain or luncheonette, attended weekly dances featuring a local orchestra, or played on the hospital baseball team, part of a state hospital league.

The hospital offered state-of-the-art treatments such as insulin coma therapy for schizophrenia, ECT, and on-site Alcoholics Anonymous (AA) meetings. In addition to treatment, the hospital strove for behavioral containment in severely ill patients. To that end, some patients were placed in warm baths. A small minority, 0.033%, were in restraints almost daily in 1932. Each month hospital administration monitored serious incidents such as deaths, escapes, fights, self-abuse, and assaults on staff. Staff often lost their jobs if patient injuries could not be adequately explained.

1.2.4 Exposés of state hospitals

Exposés of state hospitals started with conscientious objectors, known as "conchies," who were assigned alternate duty during World War II as attendants in state hospitals. There they witnessed disturbing, inhumane conditions. Their reports eventually reached members of Congress and, through the work of journalists, the general public (Torrey, 1988).

Conchies informed a 1946 *Life* magazine article (Maisel 1946) that compared state hospitals to concentration camps. The article featured several disturbing photos (e.g., one of many completely naked men in a large, unfurnished room, most crouched against a wall). Its author linked abuse and neglect to staffing practices. Attendants were unscreened, untrained, overworked, and underpaid. Physicians were assigned to care for hundreds of patients. The author briefly mentioned that conditions were better in some states where hospitals hired sufficient staff and limited their hospital populations.

Another journalist, Mike Gorman, condemned Oklahoma's state hospitals in a book *Oklahoma Attacks Its Snake Pit* (1947) that was later (in 1948) condensed in *Reader's Digest*. As Torrey (1988, p.76) wrote, "Gorman's stories mixed hyperbole and invective in a way that could hardly be ignored."

1.3 WHYS AND HOWS OF HOSPITAL CONTRACTION

1.3.1 US psychiatrists abandon the asylum

Beginning in the early 1900s, many US psychiatrists abandoned the mental illness or medical model of asylum psychiatry in favor of mental hygiene (later mental health), dynamic psychiatry, and psychoanalysis. By 1957, only 17% of American Psychiatric Association (APA) members were working in state or Veterans Affairs (VA) mental hospitals. Psychiatrists turned away from state hospitals to make their careers treating people in the community (Grob, 1994).

The mental hygiene movement began around the time hygienic measures such as purification of drinking water and aseptic technique in surgery were wildly successful in preventing infectious disease (Blevens & Bronze, 2010). The goal of mental hygiene was to prevent mental illness. Prevention was seen as possible and easier than treatment and cure.

Adolf Meyer was the most influential psychiatrist of his time and an early proponent of mental hygiene and dynamic psychiatry. Dynamic psychiatry held that clear distinctions between mental illness and health do not exist. It endorsed outpatient treatment of psychologically troubled individuals to prevent severe mental disorders (Grob, 1994).

Clifford Beers had planned to reform state hospitals but Meyer and others dissuaded him (Torrey, 1988). Beers wrote, "my plan broadened from reform to cure, from cure to prevention" (Beers, 2009, p. 128). He joined Meyer to found the National Committee for Mental Hygiene (NCMH) (Grob, 1994).

Psychoanalysis and therapies informed by psychoanalytic theory became the treatment of choice for private practitioners treating functional patients. Few US-born psychiatrists were willing to accept jobs in state hospitals, jobs that held the lowest status of all possible psychiatric employment (Torrey, 1988). State hospitals were mainly staffed by international medical graduates, many with minimal training in psychiatry (Grob, 1992).

1.3.2 Laws and court rulings lead to contraction

Psychotropic drugs had a profound effect on the practice of psychiatry, but efforts to shift treatment away from state hospitals were well under way before the efficacy of antipsychotics in chronically mentally ill adults was well understood. State hospital psychiatrists began using these drugs in the mid-1950s (see Chapter 3.2), but state and federal laws directing funds to treatment sites apart from state hospitals were enacted as early as 1946. In 1963, when President John F. Kennedy proposed funding community mental health clinics, he cited the benefits of new drugs (this a year before the publication of a report covering the first large placebo-controlled trial of antipsychotics; Guttmacher, 1964). After the wide expansion of mental health clinics and general hospital psychiatry wards began, the function of the remaining state hospital system was refashioned by court legal decisions issued mostly in the 1970s.

An early New York state law supporting treatment outside of state hospitals was the 1954 Community Mental Health Services Act. The Act reimbursed half the expenses counties or cities incurred in creating outpatient clinics, psychiatric rehabilitation services, or psychiatric wards in general hospitals. Other states followed New York's lead (Grob, 1994).

On the national level, the Hill-Burton Act of 1946 supported expansion of general hospitals, thus providing room for psychiatric wards (Grob 1994). The National Mental Health Act of 1946 provided support for research, professional training, and the establishment of community clinics, but allotted nothing for state hospitals. The Act also established the National Institute for Mental Health (NIMH). Its leader from 1949 to 1964, Dr. Robert Felix, wrote that the underlying goal of NIMH was prevention of mental illness, not the direct care and treatment of mentally ill people (Felix, 1949).

The 1955 Mental Health Study Act created a group to study US psychiatric care and treatment, the Joint Commission on Mental Illness and Health (Grob, 1994).

Dr. Felix selected a psychoanalyst, Dr. Jack R. Ewalt, to direct the work of the Commission. Another member was Mike Gorman, author of *Oklahoma Attacks Its Snake Pit* (Torrey, 1988).

The Commission's report informed President Kennedy's views when he proposed the Community Mental Health Act. He decried state hospital overcrowding and understaffing and the years-long stays of many patients while also noting that new drugs kept hospital populations from growing. He wrote that the setting of psychiatric care had moved to general hospitals and clinics and hoped that all but a small portion of people living in large institutions would be served in the community (Kennedy, 1963).

Signed October 31, 1963, the Act provided federal grants for the construction and staffing of Community Mental Health Centers (CMHCs). Congress failed to allocate enough money to expand access to clinics to all Americans because other priorities were pressing, but the Act did provide an added impetus to community-based care (Sharfstein, 2000).

Because funding for CMHCs came directly from NIMH and did not pass through state mental health officials, CMHCs were not financially obliged to care for state hospital patients. Most gave priority to less seriously ill patients who were candidates for psychotherapy. In 1975, the primary diagnosis of only 10% of patients seen in CHMCs was schizophrenia, while 21% were diagnosed with neuroses and personality disorders (Torrey, 1988).

In 1965, the year that Congress enacted Medicaid, it also enacted the Institute for Mental Diseases (IMD) exclusion to prohibit Medicaid reimbursement for the care of any patient younger than 65 in a facility with 16 or more beds in which more than half are occupied by patients whose primary diagnosis is a psychiatric illness, such as a state psychiatric hospital. Other facilities, such as nursing homes and general hospitals, could bill Medicaid for treatment and care of patients with a primary psychiatric diagnosis. Therefore, states became motivated to shift costs by discharging patients from state hospitals, which states mostly paid for, to other sites, where treatment was paid by Medicaid. (In more recent years, the IMD exclusion has loosened to permit some exceptions. Medicaid can cover costs for treatment of inpatients younger than 22 and older than 64; see 42 C.F.R. 441.13(a)(2), Prohibitions on FFP: Institutionalized individuals).

Court decisions have limited the role of state hospitals to treat and care for people who cannot live safely in the community, the role they served in the time of Anna Agnew. Decisions have also demanded more aggressive and expensive care. The *Wyatt v. Stickney* (1971) decision mandated a right to treatment and set high standards for that treatment. *Lessard v. Schmidt* (1974) restricted involuntary commitment criteria. *Rogers v. Okin* (1979) gave hospitalized psychiatric patients the right to refuse medication treatment unless a judge decides, within certain legal requirements, that involuntary treatment is necessary. Later, *Olmstead v. LC* (1999) articulated the rights of disabled people to be free of unnecessary segregation, in the least restrictive setting necessary. These legal decisions and others are described in more detail in Chapters 5.7, 6.2, 10.1, and 10.3.

1.4 HISTORY AND FUNCTIONING 1955 TO 2020

In 1966, the Medical Director of the APA, Walter Barton, surveyed the state of psychiatric services (Barton, 2000). He noted that, from 1955 to 1965, overall public psychiatric hospital population decreased by 15%, while some hospitals, including the Worcester, Massachusetts state hospital, saw a 50% decline. Meanwhile, treatment occurred elsewhere. General hospitals opened more short-stay psychiatric wards and admitted more patients with schizophrenia. Elderly individuals were often discharged from general hospital psychiatric wards to nursing homes. Clinics took on more cases, including many former state hospital patients. In 1966, at least 5–20% of patients admitted to general hospitals were transferred to state hospitals. Barton recognized a need for state hospitals but also saw that they would have to adapt to shorten their average length of stay and offer more intensive treatment programs.

Since Barton's time, in the United States as a whole, public psychiatric hospital bed capacity has continued to steadily shrink. From 1970 to 2018, public psychiatric hospital beds decreased by 84% while the US population grew by 65%. Most of this drop occurred in the 1970s and 1980s. In 1970, there were 186 beds per 100,000 population in state and county hospitals. By 1979, there were 63 beds per 100,000 population. By 1990, the number had decreased to 37 per 100,000. Decreases continued from 20 per 100,000 in 2000 to 9.6 beds per 100,000 population in 2020. The number of beds and number of patients at any one time are measures of the same thing: hospital capacity. They are not measures of the number of people treated each year because each available bed can be used multiple times per year.

More than 50 years after Barton's paper was first published, most psychiatric treatment occurred outside state hospitals. At the end of 2018, of psychiatric inpatients, 39% were in private psychiatric hospitals, 31% were in general hospitals with psychiatric units, and 26% were in state and county hospitals. State mental health systems treat far more people in outpatient settings (e.g., clinics and residences) than in hospitals. In 2020, more than 8 million people were served by state mental health systems through a variety of mental health services. Only 1.6% of those 8 million were served in hospitals.

By some measures, Barton's vision of shorter-stay and higher-quality care has been realized. On one day in 2020, almost 40,000 patients were in all US state hospitals. Over the course of that year, each bed was used an average of 3.1 times to serve 124,519 individuals. Eighty percent of state hospitals were accredited by an independent organization in 2020. Only 33% were in 1966.

Long-term custodial care of the elderly or of individuals with neurologic or developmental disorders is no longer a major function of public hospitals. In 1971, of the population of state and county hospitals across the country, 49% were diagnosed with a psychotic illness, while 24% had neurocognitive disorders, 9% developmental disability, and 7% a substance use disorder. By 2005, only 12% carried a primary (not co-occurring) diagnosis of neurocognitive disorder, developmental disability, or substance use disorder. In 1971, of the population of state and county hospitals across the country, 29% of the population were older than 65, compared to 8.8% in 2014 (Lutterman, 2022).

State and county hospitals have come to specialize in the care of involuntary and forensic patients. A patient with a forensic legal status is ordered by a court to obtain psychiatric evaluation and, often, treatment (see Chapter 7.2 for more details). The majority of these patients are admitted for evaluation of fitness to stand trial or for fitness restoration, while a small portion have been found not guilty by reason of insanity (Wik et al., 2020). In 2018, of all patients in all US public hospitals, 54% had a forensic legal status, 36% had an involuntary status, and 11% were voluntary. In that same year, 3% in private hospitals and 4% in general hospitals had a forensic status, while 47% in private hospitals and 40% in general hospitals were involuntary. The remainder were voluntary.

Data on the US public psychiatric system as a whole obscure individual state differences. In 2020, service availability varied widely between states. The number of hospitals per state varied from 23 (in New York) to 1 in 16 states, with a median of 2. The number of beds per 100,000 people ranged from 36.2 in Virginia to 2.9 in Arizona. The average was 12.1. Most states (37 of 46) offered both chronic and acute (less than 30-day) treatment, while 3 of 46 offered only acute treatment, and 6 of 46 only long-term treatment (Lutterman, 2022).

REFERENCES

42 C.F.R. 441.13(a)(2), Prohibitions on FFP: Institutionalized individuals. See page 4. Accessed November 10, 2025, from: https://www.govinfo.gov/content/pkg/CFR-2022-title42-vol4/pdf/CFR-2022-title42-vol4-part441.pdf

Adams, R. D., Victor, M., & Ropper, A. H. (1997). *Principles of Neurology Sixth Edition.* New York: McGraw-Hill.

Agnew, A. (2016). *From Under the Cloud; or, Personal Reminiscences of Insanity (1887).* Online: Wentworth Press.

Barton, W. E. (2000). Trends in community mental health programs. *Psychiatric Services* 51:611–615. Originally published September, 1966.

Beers, C. (2009). *Clifford Beers: A Mind that Found Itself.* Middletown, DE: Readaclassic.com.

Blevins, S. M. & Bronze, M. S. (2010). Robert Koch and the "golden age" of bacteriology. *International Journal of Infectious Diseases* 14(9):e744–51. doi: 10.1016/j.ijid.2009.12.003. Epub 2010 Apr 21. PMID: 20413340. 14(2010)

Dix, D. L. (1904). Memorial to the Legislature of Massachusetts, 1843. Accessed November 10, 2025, from: https://archive.org/details/memorialtolegisl00dixd/page/n3/mode/2up

Felix, R. H. (1949). Mental disorders as a public health problem. *American Journal of Psychiatry* 106:401–406.

Gollaher, D. (1995). *Voice for the Mad: The Life of Dorothea Dix.* New York: Free Press.

Gorman, M. (1947). *Oklahoma Attacks Its Snake Pits.* Norman: University of Oklahoma Press.

Gorman, M. (1948). Oklahoma attacks its snake pits. *Reader's Digest* 55(139):139–160.
Gorman, M. (1956). *Every Other Bed*. Cleveland, OH: World Publishing Company.
Grob, G. (1980). Abuse in American mental hospitals in historical perspective: Myth and reality. *International Journal of Law and Psychiatry* 3:295–310.
Grob, G. N. (1992). Mental health in America: Myths and realities. *Health Affairs* 3:8–22.
Grob, G. N. (1994). *The Mad Among Us: A History of the Care of America's Mentally Ill*. New York: Free Press.
Guttmacher, M. S. (1964). Phenothiazine treatment in acute schizophrenia: effectiveness. The National Institute of Mental Health Psychopharmacology Service Center Collaborative Study Group. *Archives of General Psychiatry* 10:246–261.
Keefe-Cooperman, K., Ulupinar, D., & Brady-Amoon, P. (2024). Rockland State Hospital: A case approach to teaching the history of psychiatry. *Teaching of Psychology*. https://doi.org/10.1177/00986283241265657
Kennedy, J. F. (1963). special message to the congress on mental illness and mental retardation. February 5, 1963. Papers of John F. Kennedy. Presidential Papers. President's Office Files. Legislative Files. Accessed November 10, 2025, from: https://www.jfklibrary.org/asset-viewer/archives/JFKPOF/052/JFKPOF-052-012
King, L. J. (2002). *From Under the Cloud at Seven Steeples 1878–1885: The Peculiarly Saddened Life of Anna Agnew at the Indiana Hospital for the Insane*. Zionsville: Guild Press of Indiana.
Kramer, M., Goldstein, H., Israel, R. H., & Johnson, N. A. (1955). *A Historical Study of the Disposition of First Admissions to a State Mental Hospital: Experience of the Warren State Hospital during the Period 1916 to 1950: Public Health Monograph Number 32*. Washington, DC: US Government Printing Office.
Lessard v. Schmidt. On remand, 379 F. Supp. 1376 (E.D. Wis. 1974).
Lutterman, R. (2022). Trends in psychiatric inpatient capacity, United States and each state, 1970–2018. Technical Assistance Collaborative Paper No. 2. Alexandria, VA: National Association of State Mental Health Program Directors. Accessed November 10, 2025, from: https://robwipond.com/wp-content/uploads/2025/02/Trends-in-Psychiatric-Inpatient-Capacity_United-States-_1970-2018_NASMHPD-2.pdf
Maisel, A. Q. (1946). Bedlam 1946: Most U. S. mental hospitals are a shame and a disgrace. *Life* May 6.
Manderscheid, R. W., Atay, J. E., & Crider, R. A. (2009). Changing trends in state psychiatric hospital use from 2002 to 2005. *Psychiatric Services* 60(1):29–34.
Olmstead v. L. C. 527 U. S. 581(1999).
Rogers v. Okin. 478 F. Supp. 1342 (D. Mass. 1979).
Sharfstein, S. S. (2000). Whatever happened to community mental health? *Psychiatric Services* 51(5):616–620.
Torrey, E. F. (1988). *Nowhere to Go: The Tragic Odyssey of the Homeless Mentally Ill*. New York: Harper & Row.
Ward, M. J. (1946). *The Snake Pit*. New York: Random House.
Wik, A., Hollen, V., & Fisher, W. A. (2020). Forensic patients in state psychiatric hospitals 1999-2016. *CNS Spectrums* 25(2):196–206.
Wyatt v. Stickney. 325 F. Supp. 781 (M.D. Ala. 1971).
Zwelling, S. S. (1985). *Quest for a Cure: The Public Hospital in Williamsburg, Virginia, 1773–1885*. Williamsburg, VA: Colonial Williamsburg Foundation.

SECTION I

Active Treatment

2

INSIGHT AND MEDICATION ADHERENCE

When psychiatrists talk about mental illness, we use a particular conceptual model, the *medical model*. When patients do not conceive of their problems in this way, we say they lack insight into their illness. This chapter reviews ways to measure insight and how insight and other factors are related to adherence. It presents three cases: a patient who gained some insight, one who had no insight but agreed to take medication anyway, and one who had his own definition of schizophrenia.

2.1 CASE A: PEOPLE WERE PICKING ON ME

2.1.1 Case

Mr. A. was a man in his early 30s who was admitted to a state hospital after he was charged with a low-level violent crime and found not fit to stand trial. Soon after he was admitted he met with his treatment team, which included a psychiatrist, social worker, nurse, psychologist, rehabilitation therapist, peer specialist, and an attendant who represented all attendants then working on the ward.

Interview

Mr. A. said he used to be a guy who was close to his family, who enjoyed hanging out with friends and listening to music, but, 5 years ago something happened to him. Now he was trying to get his life back together. What happened 5 years ago was that his neighbors started picking on him. They stole from him and left garbage in front of the door to his apartment. They had a bad falling out that threw him off balance and made him a totally different person.

The outcome of the falling out was that he got arrested. Ever since then he had problems with the system. His first contact with psychiatry was when he was first sent to a hospital. In describing that experience, he said that, for about a week, he was held and given meds that he felt were not good for him, but he took them anyway. He said his diagnosis was severe depression.

Though he had previously held steady employment in a responsible position, a job he enjoyed, he had not worked since his first arrest. Instead, he supported himself with government assistance (food stamps) and the help of his family. Because he felt that he was a burden to his family, he moved into a shelter but, at other times, lived on the streets.

A second psychiatric hospitalization, lasting 2 weeks, occurred through the efforts of police officers and shelter staff. When asked about his symptoms at the time, he said he wanted to be alone. It was too hard being in the shelter around so many strangers.

History

Records from Mr. A's fitness to stand trial exams noted that in jail he was irritable and suspicious but able to reveal that he had been hospitalized for psychiatric problems. At first he denied that he ever experienced hallucinations but later admitted that he did. At the time of his arrest he had been homeless for the previous 6 months.

Course of treatment

Mr. A. was offered and consistently accepted risperidone 3 mg at bedtime with benztropine 1 mg. On the ward, he rarely spoke, but once, when he did, he revealed that he feared someone would hurt him in his sleep. Everybody was getting on his nerves, he said. He hated the hospital.

A few weeks into his hospitalization, when Mr. A. was sitting outdoors with his rehabilitation therapist and watching others play basketball, he said he was not sick like the other patients. He needed help, but not to be in a hospital. Then he divulged that he heard voices saying they were going to kill people; once they said they would kill him. It's not good for anyone's health, he said.

When his father called, Mr. A. refused consent for his treatment team members to talk with him, though he would allow communication with his aunt. His aunt reported that, for the previous 3 years, Mr. A. had been not listening and was difficult to talk to. He wasn't making sense and blamed people for everything. But since he had been in the hospital and accepting medication, he started to sound better; he was trying to listen more.

Over time, Mr. A. occasionally paid attention in groups. Once in a while he would smile and say hello, but he still kept apart from others. He took antipsychotic medication as prescribed, though he claimed it wasn't helpful and that he would not take it.

Second interview

A month after his first interview and soon before he was discharged with a diagnosis of schizophrenia, Mr. A. sat for a second interview.

His psychiatrist asked how the hospital had helped him.

Mr. A.: The hospital helped me to be more focused on being civilized and clear-minded. The staff here, they helped me a lot. Supposedly I have a mental illness.

Psychiatrist: Do you think you have a mental illness?

Mr. A.: I disagreed with the diagnosis before I knew the symptoms, but now that I know the symptoms, I only disagree with some.

Psychiatrist: I hope you continue taking your medications. How long do you think you need them?

Mr. A.: The rest of my life. I feel better.

Psychiatrist: Why?

Mr. A.: Therapy and meds, mostly therapy.

Psychiatrist: Therapy alone is not enough.

2.1.2 Comment

Whatever benefit Mr. A. accrued from repeated short-term community hospitalizations was short-lived because he did not continue taking medication after discharge. Like many other people with severe mental illness, at least when he was admitted, Mr. A. did not believe his problems were the result of a change within himself, the onset of a mental illness. He believed his problems were due to the actions of others. However, he did come to appreciate that medication helped him. With a longer stay in a state hospital, antipsychotics could decrease his paranoia to the extent that his treatment team could develop an alliance, however tentative, and help him understand what happened to him and what he could do to help himself.

2.1.3 Note on in-hospital psychosocial treatments

For Mr. A. and other patients, hospital treatment was not just diagnosis and medication. A multidisciplinary staff offered individual therapy and a variety of therapeutic groups to fit individual patient needs, such as substance abuse counseling, stress management, trauma recovery, and psychoeducation. *Psychoeducation* is teaching about psychiatric illness: its symptoms and treatment, the risks and benefits of treatment, and the risks of no treatment. The American Psychiatric Association Practice Guideline for the Treatment of Patients with Schizophrenia recommends it (American Psychiatric Association, 2021).

The Guideline also recommend *cognitive-behavioral therapy for psychosis* (CBTp), a structured, focused therapy to help patients monitor and challenge maladaptive thinking, such as the veracity of paranoid delusions or hallucinations. Use of this therapy is limited because few clinicians are trained in its use and because patients with active, intense symptoms have difficulty participating. Supportive psychotherapy is less focused, and its methods vary between practitioners. Available evidence is strong enough to suggest its use but not to recommend it.

REFERENCE

American Psychiatric Association. (2021). *The American Psychiatric Association Practice Guideline for the Treatment of Patients with Schizophrenia* (3rd ed.). Washington, DC: American Psychiatric Association.

2.2 INSIGHT INTO PSYCHIATRIC ILLNESS

2.2.1 What is insight?

Clinicians use the mental status exam for a global, impressionistic measure of insight into having a mental illness. Researchers use scales designed to measure insight or, a popular choice, Item 12 on the Positive and Negative Syndrome Scale (PANSS) (Kay et al., 1987). Item 12 defines lack of insight as a composite of inability to recognize psychiatric illness, inability to recognize symptoms, and denial of need for treatment.

One scale for measuring insight, the Schedule for Assessing the Three Components of Insight (SAI; David, 1990), includes three subscales: recognition of illness, recognition of delusions and hallucinations as symptoms, and treatment adherence, much the same as the three components in PANSS Item 12. In the Scale to Assess Unawareness of Mental Disorder (SUMD; Amador et al., 1993), Item 1 is awareness of mental disorder. Item 1 is highly correlated with measures of insight using the mental status exam and with PANSS measures (Lincoln et al., 2007).

Lack of insight has been called *anosognosia*. "Anosognosia" can be defined by its Greek derivation, "without disease knowledge." It is so closely associated with schizophrenia that it is one of the associated features of the illness in the definition provided by the *Diagnostic and Statistical Manual of Mental Disorders* (DSM5 TR; American Psychiatric Association, 2022). But lack of insight also occurs in the course of other severe mental disorders.

2.2.2 Prevalence of poor insight

In a study of level of unawareness of illness in a group of 412 patients with severe disorders (Amador et al., 1994), 57% of those with schizophrenia had moderate to severe unawareness of having a mental illness (assessed with Item 1 of SUMD). Awareness of illness in a group of bipolar patients, who were mostly manic and severely ill, was not significantly different. But patients with major depressive disorder with and without psychotic features had significantly more awareness of illness than did the group with schizophrenia. The difference was greatest for depressed patients without psychosis.

2.2.3 The popular rating scales PANSS and BPRS

The PANSS (Kay et al., 1987) assesses positive and negative symptoms and general psychopathology. The most common positive psychotic symptoms are delusions, hallucinations, and disorganized thinking, symptoms that are not unique to schizophrenia. Negative symptoms are a prominent feature of schizophrenia. Less dramatic than positive symptoms, they are defined by diminishment of normal functions, such as emotional expression, initiative, speech output, ability to experience pleasure, and interest in social contact (American Psychiatric Association, 2022). People with schizophrenia can also experience depressive, excited, and cognitive symptoms (Kay et al., 1987).

A scale much older than the PANSS, the 18-item Brief Psychiatric Rating Scale (BPRS; Overall & Gorham, 1962), rates positive psychotic symptoms, mood, and other symptoms.

2.2.4 Can insight change?

Psychoeducation, adherence therapy, and cognitive-behavioral therapy (CBT) are psychosocial therapies designed to increase insight into illness in people with psychotic disorders. A meta-analysis (Phelan & Sigala, 2022) of 30 studies found a small but significant effect for CBT.

An analysis of the data from 40 studies of the correlation between insight and types of symptoms in patients with schizophrenia (Mintz et al., 2003) found a consistent relationship for positive symptoms. The authors concluded that insight is affected, though to a quite small degree, by the intensity of delusions and hallucinations. This suggests that insight may improve as symptoms improve.

Change in insight with time and medication has been studied with widely varying follow-up periods and very different groups of patients with schizophrenia, making results difficult to generalize. Most studies show that insight improves with time and medical treatment, more so in first-episode patients. Improvement is usually correlated with change in symptoms but only moderately or weakly.

When patients with schizophrenia were followed over a hospitalization for acute illness (Weiler et al., 2000), insight improved from admission to discharge. Insight change was modestly correlated with symptom change. In a 12-week study (Misiak et al., 2016), insight improved significantly, but significantly more in a subgroup of first-episode patients who had less insight at baseline. Over 18 months (Mohamed et al., 2008), improved insight in a group with chronic illness was associated with decreased total, positive, and negative PANSS symptoms. Improved insight was associated with increased depressive symptoms in both the above 12-week and 18-month studies. In another 12-week trial (Wiffen et al., 2010), 49% of subjects had insight at baseline, and in a 50-week trial (Gharabawi et al., 2006),

70% did. In both studies, insight significantly changed over time but minimally. In the longer study, a third of all patients improved in insight, while a fifth worsened.

In a much longer study of 131 Indian patients with schizophrenia (Saravanan et al., 2010), insight improved steadily in the 115 who could be followed for 1 year, although the relationship between change in symptoms and change in insight was weak. After 5 years, 95 of the original 131 patients could be assessed (Johnson et al., 2012). Of those, 68% were in remission. Although BPRS total scores leveled off at 6 months, insight into having a mental illness steadily increased. In those patients who remained, more insight was moderately correlated with less psychopathology (i.e., with BPRS total score and PANNS total score).

2.2.5 Patients have other explanations

In the Johnson and colleagues 2012 study, insight into having a mental illness meant acceptance of the medical or disease model. Slightly more than half of the 95 study subjects believed this model was the best explanation for their problem. The others preferred nonmedical models—of which, by far, the most common was black magic. How patients understood their psychotic experience changed over the years of the study. When first assessed many held at least one nonmedical belief. That number decreased with treatment response, then increased with stabilization.

As with the group of Indian patients, cultural factors influence how patients understand their psychotic experience (Jacob, 2014; Murri & Amore, 2018). Social factors also have a role. For example, the fear of having a socially stigmatized illness can lead people to deny diagnosis and refuse treatment (Murri & Amore, 2018). Patient explanations of psychosis can also vary with treatment response. Patients who respond well to medication may prefer a medical model, but those who respond poorly have other explanations (Jacob, 2014).

REFERENCES

Amador, X. F., Flaum, M., Andreasen, N. C., Strauss, D. H., Yale, S. A., Clark, S. C., & Gorman, J. M. (1994). Awareness of illness in schizophrenia and schizoaffective and mood disorders. *Archives of General Psychiatry* 51:826–836.

Amador, X. F., Strauss, D. H., Yale, S. A., Flaum, M. M., Endicott, J., & Gorman, J. M. (1993). Assessment of insight in psychosis. *American Journal of Psychiatry* 150(6):873–879.

American Psychiatric Association. (2022). Schizophrenia spectrum and other psychotic disorders. In *Diagnostic and Statistical Manual of Mental Disorders*, 5th ed., text revision, pp. 101–136. Washington, DC: American Psychiatric Association.

David, A. S. (1990). Insight and psychosis. *British Journal of Psychiatry* 156:798–808.

Gharabawi, G. M., Lasser, R. A., Bossie, C. A., Zhu, Y., & Amador, X. (2006). Insight and its relationship to clinical outcomes in patients with schizophrenia or

schizoaffective disorder receiving long-acting risperidone. *International Clinical Psychopharmacology* 21:233–240.
Jacob, K. S. (2014). Insight in psychosis: An independent predictor of outcome or an explanatory model of illness? *Asian Journal of Psychiatry* 11:65–71.
Johnson, S., Sathyaseelan, M., Charles, H., Jeyaseelan, V., & Jacob, K. S. (2012). Insight, psychopathology, explanatory models and outcome of schizophrenia in India a prospective 5-year cohort study. *BMC Psychiatry* 12:159.
Kay, S. R., Fiszbein, A., & Opler, L. A. (1987). The Positive and Negative Syndrome Scale for Schizophrenia (PANSS). *Schizophrenia Bulletin* 13(2):261–276.
Lincoln, T. M., Lullman, E., & Rief, W. (2007). Correlates and long-term consequences of poor insight in patients with schizophrenia: A systematic review. *Schizophrenia Bulletin* 33(6):1324–1342.
Mintz, A. R., Dobson, K. S., & Romney, D. M. (2003). Insight in schizophrenia: A meta-analysis. *Schizophrenia Research* 1:75–88.
Misiak, B., Frydecka, D., Beszlej, J. A., Moustafa, A. A., Tybura, P., Kucharska-Mazur, J. . . ., & Samochowiec, J. (2016). Effects of antipsychotics on insight in schizophrenia: Results from independent samples of first-episode and acutely relapsed patients. *International Clinical Psychopharmacology* 31:185–191.
Mohamed, S., Rosenheck, R., McEvoy, J., Swartz, M., Stroup, S., & Lieberman, J. A. (2008). Cross-sectional and longitudinal relationships between insight and attitudes toward medication and clinical outcome in chronic schizophrenia. *Schizophrenia Bulletin* 35(2):336–346.
Murri, M. B., & Amore, M. (2018). The multiple dimensions of insight in schizophrenia-spectrum disorders. *Schizophrenia Bulletin* 45(2):277–283.
Overall, J. E., & Gorham, D. R. (1962). The Brief Psychiatric Rating Scale. *Psychological Reports* 10(3):799–812.
Phelan, S., & Sigala, N. (2022). The effect of treatment on insight in psychotic disorders: A systematic review and meta-analysis. *Schizophrenia Research* 244:126–133.
Saravanan, B., Jacob, K. S., Johnson, S., Prince, M., Bhugra, D., & David, A. S. (2010). Outcome of first-episode schizophrenia in India: Longitudinal study of effect of insight and psychopathology. *British Journal of Psychiatry* 196:454–459.
Weiler, M. A., Fleisher, M. H., & McArthur-Campbell, D. (2000). Insight and symptom change in schizophrenia and other disorders. *Schizophrenia Research* 45:29–36.
Wiffen, B. D. R., Rabinowitz, J., Lex, A., & David, A. S. Correlates, change and "state or trait" properties of insight in schizophrenia. (2010). *Schizophrenia Research* 122:94–103.

2.3 CASE B: I'M PRESSING CHARGES!

2.3.1 Case

Mr. B. was a man in his early 30s, a patient at a state psychiatric hospital, who was transferred to a specialized ward for patients with hard-to-manage aggressive behavior.

Interview

Every day, his psychiatrist would tour the ward's dayroom, speaking with each patient individually. Dr. A., in a fine suit and bow tie, kept his distance, hands behind his back, and listened. Mr. B. yelled, "I'm pressing charges! It's a cover-up! They were messing with me on that ward! They sent me here to cover up for themselves!"

Mr. B. was angry all the time; angry, argumentative, suspicious, and irritable. He denied hearing voices and denied feeling sad.

History

Reports handed down from many years revealed that Mr. B. had been raised in foster homes. He had had behavior problems starting in grade school and psychiatric hospitalizations starting in his teenage years. Records revealed nothing about his life outside hospitals. They made no mention of where he lived and with whom, if he had a partner or children, or if he had been employed.

His first hospitalization, in his mid-teens, was for auditory hallucinations, delusions that his food was poisoned, mutism, and waxy flexibility. A few years later, he was treated for paranoid delusions with periods of catatonia and assaultiveness, depressed mood, suicidal ideas, and a large weight loss. Electroconvulsive therapy (ECT) brought relief. After this hospitalization came several more admissions and discharges. Typically, upon hospital release, Mr. B. would fail to attend outpatient clinic, use illicit drugs, and stop taking his prescribed medications. Readmissions were precipitated by paranoid ideas, threats, or assaults.

Course of treatment

In his first few weeks on the ward, Mr. B. made a vigorous effort to punch another patient, a man who circled the dayroom muttering about a variety of disjointed topics, including homosexuality. Mr. B. agreed that he had an anger problem but not that he needed to be where he was or to take medication. He accused Dr. A. of trying to mess him up or kill him with medication.

Dr. A. prescribed divalproex along with an antipsychotic agent, but with little effect. Mr. B. accused the attendants of talking about him or of favoring one patient over another. Much of his waking hours he spent either on the patients' communal pay phone trying to lodge complaints with lawyers or badgering other patients to get off the phone so he could get back on.

One day he was up at four in the morning trying to awaken the other men in the dorm. "They're lazy," he said, "All they do is sleep around doing nothing." Another day he fell into an escalating argument that ended when he clambered over chairs to attack another man, only to be restrained by quick-moving ward staff.

Repeatedly, Dr. A. offered lithium, but Mr. B. consistently refused. Dr. A. searched for a friendly intermediary and, with time, found one: Ms. S., a social worker who had worked with Mr. B. in the past. This kind and sympathetic woman arrived to speak with Mr. B. alone. She succeeded where his psychiatrist had failed and convinced him to take lithium.

After about 2 weeks on lithium, Mr. B.'s speech was softer and less pressured, but his mood still turned on a dime. While he continued to say he did not have a mental illness and did not need medication, he took it anyway. After 4 weeks, interactions with his doctor toggled between friendly chats and threats and accusations. After 8 weeks, Mr. B. was easily angered but quit trying to hit other patients. Finally, he returned to his regular ward on a combination of psychotropic drugs; one was lithium.

2.3.2 Comment

Mr. B. was transferred to a specialized unit because he needed more containment and supervision than regular wards provided. The ward could prevent Mr. B. from hurting other people, thanks in great part to the brave and skillful work of hospital attendants. It also created a safe space for treatment.

The toughest part of Dr. A.'s work with Mr. B. was convincing him to accept lithium. Mr. B. did not have the ability to make a rational decision about the risks and benefits of taking medication. He had no family to ask for advice. Nearly all his life he had depended on foster care, children and family services, social services, or mental health services. The trusting relationships he had were with hospital staff members, such as a warm and familiar social worker whose advice he could accept.

2.3.3 Note on use of lithium

Mr. B., like many other patients in state psychiatric hospitals, had bipolar disorder, a disorder that creates much morbidity, comorbidity, disability, and mortality (Baldessarini et al., 2007). Its treatment is often difficult and complex, especially in patients like this one with early-onset illness, many episodes, and comorbid substance abuse (Post et al., 2011). Mr. B.'s treatment using lithium was successful in that he was calmer and no longer threatening. There is evidence that this time-tested, effective, and multipurpose drug is underutilized in the United States (Post, 2018).

REFERENCES

Baldessarini, R. J., Leahy, L., Arcona, S., Gause, D., Zhang, W., & Hennen, J. (2007). Patterns of psychotropic drug prescription for U.S. patients with diagnoses of bipolar disorder. *Psychiatric Services* 58(1):85–91.

Post, R. M. (2018). The new news about lithium: An underutilized treatment in the United States. *Neuropsychopharmacology* 43:1174–1179.

Post, R. M., Leverich, G. S., Altshuler, L. I., Frye, M. A., Suppes, T., Keck, P. E. . . . & Rowem M. (2011). *International Clinical Psychopharmacology* 26(2):96–106.

2.4 ADHERENCE IN ADULTS WITH SEVERE MENTAL ILLNESS

2.4.1 Rates of adherence

Reviewers calculated average rates of nonadherence from several studies of patients with schizophrenia, most of whom were chronically ill outpatients (Lancro et al., 2002). On average, 49.5% did not usually (i.e., at least 75% of the time) take medication as prescribed. In a review of reported rates of nonadherence in patients with bipolar illness, a 50% rate was commonly reported, but estimates varied widely (Jawad et al., 2018).

2.4.2 Adherence in adults with bipolar disorder

Substance use (Leclerc et al., 2013) and abuse (Jawad et al., 2018) are consistently and strongly associated with adherence to medication in cross-sectional studies of people with bipolar disorder. Insight into illness is not consistently correlated with adherence in this group, but a negative attitude toward medication is (Jawad et al., 2018; Leclerc et al., 2013). Patients report that weight gain and cognitive effects affect adherence (Johnson et al., 2007), as does a positive therapeutic alliance (Zeber et al., 2008).

In longitudinal studies, insight can predict medication adherence, but so can other factors such as work impairment, more psychotic symptoms, and cannabis use (Gonzalez-Pinto et al., 2010). Patient-reported current adherence is a strong predictor of future adherence (Johnson et al., 2007).

2.4.3 Adherence in adults with schizophrenia

Past adherence

Past adherence is a powerful predictor in people with schizophrenia (Novick et al., 2010; Olfson et al., 2000). In a large 3-year study of routine clinical care (Ascher-Svanum et al., 2006a), past adherence was a strong predictor of future adherence, but nonadherence was a weak predictor of nonadherence. Sixty-two percent of patients who were adherent in the first year stayed adherent in both the second and third years of the study. Of patients who were nonadherent in the first year, many became adherent. Thirty-nine percent became adherent in the second year, 37% were adherent in the third, and 24% were adherent in both years.

Illicit drugs and alcohol

In cross-sectional studies, substance abuse (Fenton et al., 1997; Lancro et al., 2002) and use (Czobor et al., 2015) are associated with nonadherence. Drug or alcohol use (Ascher-Svanum et al., 2006b) or abuse (Novick et al., 2010) also predicted nonadherence at least 1 year after use or abuse was detected. In a study of 42 individuals with schizophrenia (Pristach & Smith, 1990), most reported drinking in the month before they were admitted to hospital. Sixty-two percent of the 42 reported stopping prescribed medication while drinking. They often explained that they were told not to mix medication and alcohol.

Medication effects

Adverse effects of medication as measured by investigators are inconsistently related to noncompliance in cross-sectional studies (Czobor et al., 2015; Lancro et al., 2002; Sendt et al., 2014). One group (Robinson et al., 2002) found that parkinsonian adverse effects increased the likelihood of stopping medication, but another (Lindenmayer et al., 2009) did not find that medication tolerability and weight gain predicted stopping medication.

Adverse effects as reported by patients differed. In one survey (Weiden et al., 2004), patients disclosed that they stopped due to obesity and distress due to weight gain and, in another (DiBonaventura et al., 2012), that they stopped due to various adverse effects including extra-pyramidal symptoms, sedation, cognitive slowing, and metabolic side effects.

On the other hand, in a drug trial (Lindenmayer et al., 2009), medication beneficial effects as measured by investigators (i.e., a decrease in symptoms at any assessment) did not predict accepting treatment at the following assessment.

Aspects of schizophrenic illness

Adherence in groups of people with schizophrenia is often related to overall symptom severity (Fenton et al., 1997; Novick et al., 2010; Sendt et al., 2014). For example, in a cross-sectional study of 262 patients in routine clinical care (Bitter et al., 2015), adherence rated by treating clinicians was significantly and strongly correlated to a global impression of illness. Patients who were more ill were less adherent, and less-adherent patients were more ill.

Individual symptoms have also been related. Level of hostility was correlated with nonadherence in clinical care (Bitter et al., 2015) and in two large drug treatment studies (Czobor et al., 2015). Depressive symptoms were more likely in outpatients who reported they were not consistent in taking medications as prescribed compared to patients who said they were (Elbogen et al., 2005).

Insight

Cross-sectional studies often find a relationship between insight and adherence (Lincoln et al., 2007). For example, in an analysis of large drug trials (Czobor et al., 2015), impaired insight as measured by the Positive and Negative Syndrome Scale (PANSS) Item 12 (Kay et al., 1987) was significantly related to poor adherence. In an observational study (Bitter et al., 2015), adherence was significantly correlated with a global measure of insight (i.e., total score on the Schedule for Assessing the Three Components of Insight [SAI]; David, 1990), but a stronger correlation was found with scores on the SAI treatment adherence subscale.

Longitudinal studies have less definitive results. In Czobor and colleague's analysis (2015), impaired insight measured by PANSS Item 12 predicted poor adherence at 6 and 12 months. Among inpatients (Olfson, 2000), awareness of symptoms predicted self-reported adherence 3 months after hospital discharge, but insight into having an illness did not.

Another group (Kim et al., 2020) found that insight measured by PANSS Item 12 was a predictor of adherence, but not a robust one. Thirty-one percent of the group with good insight at the start of the study were nonadherent 18 months later, while 37% of those with fair insight and 43% with little to no insight were nonadherent.

Results of cross-sectional studies can differ from longitudinal ones because, over time, other factors come into play, such as substance abuse or use of long-acting injectables. Some studies have found that insight predicts adherence only in patients who do not abuse illicit drugs (Lincoln et al., 2007).

Attitude toward medication

One review (Sendt et al., 2014) concluded that insight and attitude toward medication were the only two factors consistently associated with better adherence. Attitude toward medication is closely related to part of the PANSS Item 12 concept of insight: insight into need for treatment.

A positive attitude toward medication or need for treatment may be more predictive than insight into illness. The Rating of Medication Influences (ROMI) scale (Weiden et al., 1994) measures patient beliefs about treatment. These include denial of having an illness and of needing medication, negative aspects of medication, perceived benefit, positive external influence, fulfillment of life goals, and stigma. In a study of the predictive value of these patient beliefs (Liu-Seifert et al., 2007), a higher level of perceived benefit was the only factor that significantly predicted less likelihood of antipsychotic discontinuation over 12 months.

2.4.4 Strategies to improve adherence

The above review can guide clinicians as they meet with individual patients to explore their past experience with medication, try to understand why they have or have not taken it, and learn what they think and feel about taking medication in the future. A direct discussion can identify and address factors that have been associated with nonadherence. It can reveal patients' attitudes about medication and encourage them to articulate how they think it either could help them in the future or cause more difficulties.

A psychiatric researcher and dedicated practitioner (Fenton et al., 1997) advised an approach to such discussions and to treatment in general. To summarize, he emphasized using a negotiated, nonauthoritarian approach and encouraging open discussion of deviation from the clinician's recommendations. He advised understanding the patient and his or her concerns and goals, centering the treatment on helping the patient attain his or her goals, and communicating hope that meeting at least one goal is possible. That goal should be attainable and important to the patient, and may not be remission.

A patient is more likely to follow a simple regimen. Once-, or at most, twice-daily dosing of oral medication is preferable, with the minimum number of prescriptions and the minimum number of pills. A long-acting injectable is the simplest regimen and superior for preventing relapse (see Chapter 3.6).

REFERENCES

Ascher-Svanum, H., Faries, D. E., Zhu, B., Ernst, F. R., Swartz, M. S., & Swanson, W. (2006a). Medication adherence and long-term functional outcomes in the treatment of schizophrenia in usual care. *Journal of Clinical Psychiatry* 67:453–460.

Ascher-Svanum, H., Zhu, B., Faries, D., Lancro, J. P., & Dolder, C. R. (2006b). A prospective study of risk factors for nonadherence with antipsychotic medication in the treatment of schizophrenia. *Journal of Clinical Psychiatry* 67:1114–1123.

Bitter, I., Feher, L., Tenyi, T., & Czobor, P. (2015). Treatment adherence and insight in schizophrenia. *Psychiatria Hungarica* 30 (1):18–26.

Czobor, P., Van Dorn, R. A., Citrome, L., Kahn, R. S., Fleischkacker, W. W., & Volavka, J. (2015). Treatment adherence in schizophrenia: A patient-level meta-analysis of combined CATIE and EUFEST studies. *European Neuropsychopharmacology* 25(8):1158–1166.

David, A. S. (1990). Insight and psychosis. *British Journal of Psychiatry* 156:798–808.

DiBonaventura, M., Gabriel, S., Dupclay, L., Gupta, S., & Kim, E. (2012). A patient perspective on the impact of medication side effects on adherence: Results of a cross-sectional nationwide survey of patients with schizophrenia. *BMC Psychiatry* 20(12):20. doi: 10.1186/1471-244X-12-20. PMID: 22433036; PMCID: PMC3342101.

Elbogen, E. B., Swanson, J. W., Swartz, M. S., & Van Dorn, R. (2005). Medication nonadherence and substance abuse in psychotic disorders: Impact of depressive symptoms and social stability. *Journal of Nervous and Mental Disorders* 193(10):673–679.

Fenton, W. S., Blyler, C. R., & Heinssen, R. K. (1997). Determinants of medication compliance in schizophrenia: Empirical and clinician findings. *Schizophrenia Bulletin* 23(4):637–651.

Gonzalez-Pinto, A., Reed, C., Novick, D., Bertsch, J., & Haro, J. M. (2010). Assessment of medication adherence in a cohort of patients with bipolar disorder. *Pharmacopsychiatry* 43:263–270.

Jawad, I., Watson, S., Haddad, P. M., Talbot, P. S., & McAllister-Williams, R. H. (2018). Medication nonadherence in bipolar disorder: A narrative review. *Therapeutic Advances in Psychopharmacology* 8(12):349–363.

Johnson, F. R., Ozdemir, S., Manjunath, R., Hauber, A. B., Burch, S. P., & Thompson, R. (2007). Factors that affect adherence to bipolar treatments: a stated-preference approach. *Medical Care* 45(6):545–552.

Kay, S. R., Fiszbein, A., & Opler, L. A. (1987). The Positive and Negative Syndrome Scale for Schizophrenia (PANSS). *Schizophrenia Bulletin* 13(2):261–276.

Kim, J., Ozzoude, M., Nakajima, S., Shah, P., Caravaggio, F., Itawa, Y., . . . & Gerretsen, P. (2020). Insight and medication adherence in schizophrenia: An analysis of the CATIE trial. *Neuropharmacology* 68(168):107634. doi: 10.1016/j.neuropharm.2019.05.011. Epub 2019 May 9. PMID: 31077729.

Lancro, J. P., Dunn, L. B., Dolder, C. R., Dunn, L. B., Dolder, C. R., Leckband, S. G., & Jeste, D. V. (2002). Prevalence of and risk factors for medication nonadherence in patients with schizophrenia: A comprehensive review of recent literature. *Journal of Clinical Psychiatry* 63:892–909.

Leclerc, E., Mansur, R. B., & Brietzke, E. (2013). Determinants of adherence in bipolar disorder: A comprehensive review. *Journal of Affective Disorders* 149:247–252.

Lincoln, T. M., Lullman, E., & Rief, W. (2007). Correlates and long-term consequences of poor insight in patients with schizophrenia: A systematic review. *Schizophrenia Bulletin* 33(6):1324–1342.

Lindenmayer, J. P., Liu-Seifert, H., Kulkarni, P. M., Kinon, B. J., Stauffer, V., Edwards, S. E., . . . & Volavka, J. (2009). Medication nonadherence and treatment outcome in patients with schizophrenia or schizoaffective disorder with suboptimal prior response. *Journal of Clinical Psychiatry* 70(7):990–996.

Liu-Seifert, H., Adams, D. H., Ascher-Svanum, H., Faries, D. E., & Kinon, B. J. (2007). Patient perception of medication benefit and early treatment discontinuation in a 1-year study of patients with schizophrenia. *Patient Prefer Adherence* 1:9–17. PMID: 19956443; PMCID: PMC2779124.

Novick, D., Haro, J. M., Suarez, D., Perez, V., Dittman, R. W., & Haddad, P. M. (2010). Predictors and clinical consequences of non-adherence with antipsychotic medication in the outpatient treatment of schizophrenia. *Psychiatry Research* 176:109–113.

Olfson, M., Mechanic, D., Hansell, S., Boyer, C. A., Walkup, J., & Weiden, P. J. (2000). Predicting medication noncompliance after hospital discharge among patients with schizophrenia. *Psychiatric Services* 51(2):216–222.

Pristach, C. A., & Smith, C. M. (1990). Medication compliance and substance abuse among schizophrenic patients. *Hospital and Community Psychiatry* 41(12):1345–1348.

Robinson, D. G., Woerner, M. G., Alvir, J. M. J., Bilder, R. M., Hinrichsen, G. A., & Lieberman, J. A. (2002). Predictors of medication discontinuation by patients with first-episode schizophrenia and schizoaffective disorder. *Schizophrenia Research* 57(2-3):209–219.

Sendt, K. V., Tracy, D. K., & Bhattacharyya, S. (2014). A systematic review of factors influencing adherence to antipsychotic medication in schizophrenia-spectrum disorders. *Psychiatry Research* 225:14–30.

Weiden, P., Rapkin, B., Mott, T., Zygmunt, A., Goldman, D., Horvitz-Lennon, M., & Francis, A (1994). Rating of medication influences (ROMI) scale in schizophrenia. *Schizophrenia Bulletin* 20:297–310.

Weiden, P. J., Mackell, J. A., & McDonnell, D. D. (2004). Obesity as a risk factor for antipsychotic compliance. *Schizophrenia Research* 66(1):51–57.

Zeber, J. E., Copeland, L. A., Good, C. B., Fine, M. J., Bauer, M. S., & Kilbourne, A. M. (2008). Therapeutic alliance perceptions and medication adherence in patients with bipolar disorder. *Journal of Affective Disorders* 107(1-3):53–62.

2.5 CASE C: I'M TRYING TO REGAIN A PROGRAM FOR MY LIFE

2.5.1 Case

Mr. C. was a patient in his early 50s who was admitted to a state psychiatric hospital after he was arrested, charged with a misdemeanor violent crime, and found not fit to stand trial. His charges were dropped. Treatment with antipsychotic medication brought his symptoms into remission, so his treatment team started preparing discharge plans. A first step was to get a second opinion. He was interviewed by an in-hospital consulting team of a social worker and a psychiatrist to clear him for discharge.

Interview

Social Worker: What was going on with you before you were arrested?
Mr. C.: My main problem was alcohol. I had lost strength and concentration. I was drinking daily and taking long walks. It wasn't healthy. On the streets, I dropped my guard and was living in a fantasy world. I wasn't living responsible. I drank to get away from hard times. But drinking is not the way to get away from reality.

Mr. C. admitted to the crime for which he was arrested and expressed regret.

Psychiatrist: What are your plans for the future?
Mr. C.: I want to go to AA meetings. I want to participate with some sober minds and gain some strength, to have someone to relate to. I want to refrain from the drinking life. I'm too old. I'm trying to regain a program for my life.
Psychiatrist: What does your medication do for you?
Mr. C.: It gives me a security as far as my illness is concerned.
Psychiatrist: And what is that illness?
Mr. C.: Schizophrenia.
Psychiatrist: What does that mean?
Mr. C.: It's hard to explain. I have a personality conflict; I'm in conflict with myself. I want my personality to fit society.

History

Mr. C.'s life was going smoothly; he had a job, a wife, and children. But, in his early 20s, he became paranoid about his co-workers and soon was unable to work. A few early hospitalizations were followed by many years out of hospitals during which he attended outpatient clinics and lived with his family. When his wife died, he sometimes turned to his sister, but more often to the streets, shelters, and heavy alcohol use.

2.5.2 Comment

Mr. C. had his own way of explaining the problems that brought him to the hospital and what medication did for him. He knew what he needed to do to keep safe in the future. His psychiatrist did not need to instruct him on symptoms, brain dysfunction, or the medical model.

3

ANTIPSYCHOTIC TREATMENT

This chapter explores how people with schizophrenia benefit when they take antipsychotic drugs consistently. It also includes a brief comparison of antipsychotic drugs and suggestions for prescribing. In three case histories, one patient has an excellent short-term symptomatic response, one has a partial response, and one achieved symptomatic remission with a change in antipsychotic agent.

3.1 CASE D: I'M A VICTIM OF RACIAL DISCRIMINATION

3.1.1 Case

Ms. D. was a woman in her early 60s, a member of an ethnic minority. She was admitted to a state hospital after she was charged with a low-level crime and found not fit to stand trial.

INTERVIEW

Soon after admission Ms. D. told her treatment team that her most urgent concern was back and leg pain. "I am crippled," she said, though everyone could see that she walked without difficulty.

Her psychiatrist asked why she couldn't work, why, after helping to support her family for years, she quit. Being crippled was one reason, but another was stalking and harassment. She claimed she was a victim of racial discrimination, that everywhere she went people stalked and harassed her. They elbowed her, they approached her in public places, and taunted her with racial slurs. Her alleged crime was the outcome of such an encounter. She believed the police were part of the conspiracy against her. Fears of stalking affected her ability to leave her home to work and shop. Her psychiatrist asked if she thought these problems could be in her mind. Her response was "No. See the evidence."

Her team also talked about her treatment. Aripiprazole hit her hard, she said, and she asked for a lower dose. Another drug she had taken in the past caused sore eyes. But she agreed to take the medication once she got home, if her psychiatrist wanted her to.

History

Until 3 years before her state hospital admission, Ms. D. had never been in psychiatric treatment or arrested. She was a lucky woman, with a home, a devoted spouse, and two grown children. Her husband told the team's social worker that after Ms. D. watched her mother deteriorate and die after a long illness, his wife was not the same in that she stopped working and developed pain. Twice in the previous 3 years she was arrested after she defended herself from delusional persecutors; both times she was found not fit to stand trial due to psychiatric illness. After two previous arrests she was sent from jail to an emergency room, where she was prescribed an antipsychotic drug that she did not take more than once or twice. Her third arrest resulted in her current hospitalization.

Course of treatment

On admission, Ms. D. had complete physical, neurological, and cognitive exams—all unremarkable. An internist found no physical cause for her complaints of pain. After 3 or 4 weeks of aripiprazole 10 mg daily, her physical complaints stopped. On the other hand, she still believed in the conspiracy. When asked, she said she could ignore the stalkers but could not return to work, not right away.

Another 4 weeks and an increase in aripiprazole to 25 mg brought an amazing reversal. She was fine, she said, she was being treated like family in our hospital. Her lawyer had sent her to us for treatment, which had been very good. The medication and the program were designed to help her.

Her psychiatrist asked if she was worried about people following her, as she had been. She said that was more like a delusion . . . imaginary. Ms. D. expected no such troubles when she left the hospital, just as she had had none in the hospital. She missed her husband and children and was eager to go home and see them again. Family visits had been difficult because her husband had been holding two jobs to support their family. She wanted to get back to work.

3.1.2 Comment

For Ms. D., an emergency room visit, a prescription, and an appointment at an outpatient clinic did not prevent another arrest. In a hospital, it took several weeks—not days—to convince her to accept a therapeutic dose of medication and for it to become effective enough that she could abandon her delusions. This woman was unusual in her insight and full response to treatment without discernible symptoms and with the ability to return to her family and job.

3.1.3 Note on predictors of symptomatic remission

This patient did not meet the current *Diagnostic and Statistical Manual of Mental Disorders* (DSM-5 TR) criteria for schizophrenia because she had only delusions (American Psychiatric Association, 2022). To meet criteria requires additional symptoms: either hallucinations, disorganized speech or behavior, or negative symptoms. Her history and the characteristics of her illness are predictors of a remitting psychotic illness (see Chapter 3.4).

REFERENCE

American Psychiatric Association. (2022). *Diagnostic and Statistical Manual of Mental Disorders* (5th ed. text revision).Washington, DC: American Psychiatric Publishing.

3.2 EARLY EXPERIENCE WITH ANTIPSYCHOTICS

3.2.1 Early reports of clinical use

The first antipsychotic to reach a broad market was chlorpromazine. Mid-1950s inpatient psychiatrists gave it glowing reviews. One (Kinross-Wright, 1955) wrote "the total sedative requirements for the service have been greatly reduced since this new treatment was instituted. Also worth mentioning is the strange, striking quiet which has come over the ward with its population of acutely disturbed patients." Another (Cowden et al., 1956) wrote, "The drug appears to have its greatest value in quieting disturbed, anxious patients and making them amenable to other therapies."

Early on, psychiatrists did not know which patients would most benefit from chlorpromazine. They did not know it was an antipsychotic. They described its use in groups of patients with a mixed bag of diagnoses—schizophrenia, depression, anxiety states, and others—in both state hospitals and on the psychiatric units of general hospitals. One group studied the use of chlorpromazine as an adjunct to group psychotherapy (Cowden et al., 1956). Investigators described particularly gratifying results with schizophrenic patients (Kinross-Wright, 1955). It was noted early on that chlorpromazine treatment of less chronic, younger patients with schizophrenia was more successful than treatment of more chronic patients (Feldman, 1957).

3.2.2 A placebo-controlled trial of efficacy

The year 1964 brought the publication of a landmark study of the efficacy of three antipsychotic drugs (chlorpromazine, fluphenazine, and thioridazine) versus placebo in the treatment of adults with schizophrenia (Guttmacher, 1964). This was a short-term study of the use of drugs then available in treating acutely ill individuals. All 344 patients completing the 6-week study were newly admitted inpatients. Half were suffering from their first psychotic episode. Almost all (82%) were at least markedly ill at the start of the study.

Diagnostic criteria were not specified. To understand how patients changed over 6 weeks of treatment, researchers made global assessments of severity of mental illness (rated from (1) normal, to (7) among the most extremely ill) and of improvement (rated from (1) very much improved, to (7) very much worse). They also measured individual symptoms and ward behavior.

The authors concluded that the three drugs had many actions in addition to quieting excited patients. Although the three antipsychotic drugs tested differed in incidence of multiple adverse effects, there was no significant difference in patient benefits so measurement of benefits for all drugs was lumped together.

In the global assessment of severity of illness, the median rating for the drug-treated group was (3), mildly ill, while the median rating for the placebo-treated group was between (4) moderately ill and (5) markedly ill.

In the global improvement assessment, the difference between drug- and placebo-treated patients was highly significant. Almost all (95%) of drug-treated patients were rated as improved, 75% either (1) very much or (2) much improved. Only 5% showed no change. The median degree of improvement for drug-treated patients was rated as (2), much improved, and for placebo patients (3), minimally improved. Analysis of trends showed that clinical change probably did not plateau at 6 weeks.

Investigators found a significant difference between placebo and active treatment groups in several symptoms including hostility, disorientation, auditory hallucinations, agitation and tension, slowed speech and movements, indifference to environment, incoherent speech, and ideas of persecution. They also found significant differences in behavioral measures including social participation, self-care, confusion, and irritability.

3.2.3 Placebo-controlled trials 1955–2016

A 2017 publication reviewed 67 trials from 1955 to 2016 comparing antipsychotic drugs (but not clozapine or long-acting injectables) to placebo (Leucht et al., 2017). Twenty-eight thousand patients with schizophrenia and closely related disorders were participants in these trials.

Good response was defined as at least much improved on a global assessment or at least a 50% reduction in ratings on the Brief Psychiatric Rating Scale (BPRS) (Overall & Gorham, 1962) or the Positive and Negative Syndrome Scale (PANNS) (Kay et al., 1987). A minimal response was defined as at least minimally improved on a global assessment or a more than 20% reduction in ratings on BPRS or PANNS.

In this review, 23% of drug-treated patients showed a good response, as did 14% of placebo-treated patients. Fifty-one percent of drug-treated patients showed at least a minimal response compared to 30% of patients on placebo.

The review reached additional conclusions: drug treatment was more effective in alleviating positive symptoms than negative or depressive symptoms. Drug-treated patients had better social functioning and quality of life. Antipsychotic drugs had significantly more adverse effects compared to placebo.

The methods used in the 1964 Guttmacher study differ from trials analyzed by Leucht and others in ways that could influence their results. The studies differed in diagnostic criteria. In more recent years, investigators use standard diagnostic criteria, which are probably more restrictive than those used in 1964. The studies differed in psychopathology ratings. The review reported on symptom improvement measured by standardized rating scales. The 1964 study used global assessments and a rating scale that is now out of use. The most important difference was in choice of participants. Unlike the 1964 study, none of the 67 trials was restricted to first-episode patients; their participants were predominantly chronically ill, often previously treated people. In addition, people with schizophrenia who volunteered for these trials are an unrepresentative group who may be more likely to be only partial responders or placebo responders (Leucht et al., 2017).

REFERENCES

Cowden, R. C., Zax, A. M., Hague, J. R. & Finney, R. C. (1956). Chlorpromazine: Alone and as adjunct to group psychotherapy in the treatment of psychiatric patients. *American Journal of Psychiatry* 112(11):898–902.

Feldman, P. E. (1957). Two-year fate study of Thorazine-treated patients. *American Journal of Psychiatry* 114(3):237–240.

Guttmacher, M. S. (1964). Phenothiazine treatment in acute schizophrenia: Effectiveness. The National Institute of Mental Health Psychopharmacology Service Center Collaborative Study Group. *Archives of General Psychiatry* 10:246–261.

Kay, S. R., Fiszbein, A., & Opler, L. A. (1987). The Positive and Negative Syndrome Scale (PANNS) for schizophrenia. *Schizophrenia Bulletin* 13:261–276.

Kinross-Wright, V. (1955). Chlorpromazine treatment of mental disorders. *American Journal of Psychiatry* 111(12):907–912.

Leucht, S., Leucht, C., Huhn, M., Chaimani, A., Mavridis, D., Helfer, B., . . . & Davis, J. M. (2017). Sixty years of placebo-controlled antipsychotic drug trial in acute schizophrenia: Systematic review, Bayesian meta-analysis, and meta-regression of efficacy predictors. *American Journal of Psychiatry* 10:927–942.

Overall, J. E., & Gorham, D. R. (1962). The Brief Psychiatric Rating Scale. *Psychological Reports* 10:790–812.

3.3 CASE E: NO! NEVER! I'M NOT PSYCHOTIC!

3.3.1 Case

Mr. E. was a young man who was charged with a felony and found not fit to stand trial. He was admitted to a state psychiatric hospital for restoration of fitness.

Interview

A few days after Mr. E. arrived at the hospital, he punched another patient and injured an attendant who intervened. The next day, two attendants escorted the young man into a conference room and stood attentively, one behind each shoulder, as he met with his treatment team.

His psychiatrist asked what happened between him and the other patient.

Mr. E.: He kept staring at me, giving me dirty looks, calling me a pussy and a punk. I'm being abused.
Psychiatrist: What about the other patient?
Mr. E.: He was looking at me and laughing. He was frowning and provoking me in the bathroom.
Psychiatrist: Are you taking your meds?
Mr. E.: Yes. And I go to class every day. I want to study aviation.

His social worker pointed out that people were injured.

Mr. E.: They punched me! I'm not sick!

The social worker told him he was in a hospital, a place with rules, where he should listen to what staff told him.

Mr. E.: They verbally abuse me! They provoke me!

History

Fitness examiners who interviewed Mr. E. in jail reported that he was smelly, suspicious, irritable, and angry. Rather than talk about his charges, he was preoccupied with complaints that he was threatened and taunted by the man housed next to him. Mr. E. disclosed little except that he lived with his parents, was not working, and did not use alcohol or illicit drugs. Examiners knew that he had been hospitalized the year before because his mother had so informed his lawyer and his lawyer informed the examiners. Mr. E. denied it, saying, "No! Never! I'm not psychotic! I'm not a danger to myself or others!" Because he refused consent to allow access to his psychiatric records, examiners could not research his history.

Second interview

The next day Mr. E. was still incensed by perceived harassment by other patients. After he punched another attendant in the process of being restrained, he was transferred to a small ward with more supervision. He came into the conference room, shook hands with those near him, then sat still, with his hands folded, looking down during most of the interview.

Psychiatrist: How are you?
Mr. E.: I'm doing great.
Psychiatrist: What happened on the other ward?
Mr. E.: Nothing special.

PSYCHIATRIST: You mean you didn't hit people?

MR. E.: That was a misunderstanding.

PSYCHIATRIST: Do you know why you are here? Do you know you need medicine for your brain to work well? That you have a psychiatric problem? Has anyone told you that?

MR. E.: No.

PSYCHIATRIST: Why have you been getting into psychiatric hospitals?

MR. E.: I dunno.

PSYCHIATRIST: This is a psychiatric hospital. Do you know what you have to do in a psychiatric hospital?

MR. E.: Take my medicine.

COURSE OF TREATMENT

On his new ward, Mr. E. approached attendants who were not addressing him, asked their names, and then called into a complaint line to report they were berating him, planning to hurt him, or asking for sexual favors. They did none of these things. He was hallucinating and paranoid. When ward staff asked how he was doing, he threatened to report them for harassment. He would not allow a social worker to talk with his family and would not reveal where he was previously hospitalized.

After a few weeks of accepting medication regularly, Mr. E. said it helped him feel calmer, though he also said he didn't need it because he had no mental illness, that he only took it to get out of the hospital. His calls to the complaint line stopped. He could focus on conversations and keep himself clean, ask for what he needed, and participate in groups. Even so, he was still paranoid. When asked what he was stuffing into his sock, he said he was being harassed, so he had a pen next to him to be safe. Because he never disclosed any family phone numbers, his mother remained in the dark, without knowledge of his treatment. And he insisted fighting was not his fault—not at all: it was reasonable.

This young man was eventually returned to court to face his charges. In court, Mr. E. agreed to participate in an alternatives to incarceration program, a program that would refer him to treatment and other services, perhaps housing, and keep a close eye on him. As long as he met its requirements, he could avoid jail or prison time. See Chapter 11.2 for another case of a man referred to an alternatives to incarceration program.

3.3.2 Comment

Mr. E. was treated with antipsychotic medication in a setting that contained and curtailed his ongoing violent behavior, another testament to the dedication of state hospital ward staff. It was his bad luck, like that of many patients, that he had an incomplete response. His paranoia abated but remained. More important for his psychiatrist's decision to discharge, his functioning improved in that he quit punching others, quit complaining that people were talking about him, and could listen and talk reasonably with others. If he continued taking medication, whether he believed he needed it or not, he had a chance of staying relatively well and out of jail.

3.4 OUTCOMES OF TREATMENT WITH ANTIPSYCHOTICS

A placebo-controlled trial gives an idea of how antipsychotics can affect symptoms over weeks. Like Mr. E., many patients have an incomplete, short-term response. Other, broader measures demonstrate how and how much these drugs improve patients' lives over months and years.

3.4.1 Symptomatic remission

Symptomatic remission is more than response; it is having a minimally severe illness for a defined duration of time. A consensus definition of symptomatic remission for schizophrenia from the Remission in Schizophrenia Working Group (RSWG) includes criteria for severity of three groups of symptoms as well as a time threshold (Andreasen et al., 2005). The groups of symptoms are delusions and hallucinations, disorganization of speech and behavior, and negative symptoms. These symptoms must be absent or at a mild level using the Brief Psychiatric Rating Scale (BPRS; Overall & Gorham, 1962) or Positive and Negative Syndrome Scale (PANSS; Kay et al., 1987) for at least 6months.

Although rates are variable, a substantial proportion of patients achieve remission at some time during the course of their illness. Rates can vary according to duration of follow-up, medication adherence, and type of treatment (Ventura et al., 2011). A review of studies that followed first- and multi-episode patients for at least 6 months but up to 5 years (Lambert et al., 2010) concluded that, on average across studies, 40% of patients were lost to follow-up. Those who dropped out were less likely to have achieved remission. Forty-eight percent of first-episode study completers met full RSWG remission criteria at some point in the follow-up period, while 43% of multi-episode completers did so.

Level of functioning before treatment (Carbon & Correll, 2014; van Dee et al., 2023) or before illness onset (Carbon & Correll, 2014; Lambert et al., 2010) is a powerful predictor of remission. History of childhood trauma (van Dee et al., 2023) and substance abuse that persists past the start of treatment predict non-remission.

Less-chronic illness predicts remission, where less chronicity is manifested by first-episode illness, fewer previous hospital admissions (van Dee et al., 2023), fewer relapses, and shorter illness duration (Carbon & Correll, 2014). Less overall psychopathology (Carbon & Correll, 2014; Lambert et al., 2010; van Dee et al., 2023) and, in particular, less severe negative symptoms predict remission (Carbon & Correll, 2014).

Some aspects of treatment predict non-remission. Duration of untreated psychosis (Lambert et al., 2010; van Dee et al., 2023) is a significant predictor even after controlling for poor premorbid adjustment (Carbon & Correll, 2014). Lack of early antipsychotic benefits is also predictive, as is, to a lesser degree, early adverse effects (Carbon & Correll 2014).

3.4.2 Recovery and other types of remission

Other important aspects of outcome are functioning and well-being. In one study, patients preferred subjective well-being, but psychiatrists preferred symptom decrease (Karow et al., 2012). *Functional remission* is often defined as a span of 6 months of adequate functioning in employment, social contacts, and independent living. *Well-being remission* is 6 months of satisfaction in life. Recovery is a higher bar to reach. Recovery often requires at least 2 years of symptomatic, functional, and well-being remission, although it does not have a broadly accepted definition (Lambert et al., 2008).

A study of 2,960 individuals with schizophrenia, most of whom were chronically ill, determined rates of remission (Lambert et al., 2006). During some span of 6 months within a 2-year follow-up, 47% of patients met criteria for symptomatic remission, 42% for well-being remission, and 27% for functional remission. Only 13% were at some time in remission in all three spheres, while 35% were never in remission in any. Obtaining employment was the greatest obstacle to attaining complete remission. Without this criteria, 23% would have been in remission in all three spheres at some time in 2 years.

Recovery in all three outcomes is uncommon even in nonchronic patients. A study that followed 392 acutely ill, never before treated people with schizophrenia over 3 years, found that only 17% had achieved full recovery during some span of 24 months (Lambert et al., 2008).

3.4.3 Outcomes of adherence versus nonadherence

Another way to evaluate the value of antipsychotic medication is to compare outcomes in patients who take it to outcomes in patients who do not.

Taking medication as prescribed does not always prevent relapse but makes it less likely. An analysis of 65 studies compared continuing antipsychotic medication to stopping. After 1 year, 64% of patients on placebo had relapsed compared to 27% of those on active drugs (Leucht et al., 2012). A 3-year study (Caseiro et al., 2012) tracked 140 first-episode patients whose symptoms were improved and stable. Over 3 years, 65% of the entire group relapsed at least once, but 94% of the nonadherent group relapsed compared to 50% of adherent patients. On average, nonadherent patients relapsed more quickly.

In multiple studies, nonadherent patients had more hospitalizations (Ascher-Svanum et al., 2006; Novick et al., 2010; Olfson et al., 2000), more emergency room use (Ascher-Svanum et al., 2006; Olfson et al., 2000), more symptoms, a greater likelihood of homelessness (Olfson et al., 2000), and a greater likelihood of suicide attempts (Novick et al., 2010) compared to adherent patients.

Adherent patients had better functioning and life satisfaction in a study of 1,906 individuals with schizophrenia followed for 3 years (Ascher-Svanum et al., 2006). Those who took medication consistently in the first study year had significant and lasting improvements in the next 2 years in mental functioning, satisfaction of basic needs, and life in general compared to those who were inconsistent. The difference between groups was mostly due to improvement in the adherent group but also to worsening in the nonadherent group. Nonadherent patients were more likely to be arrested even if they had never been arrested before the study began.

Use of antipsychotic drugs in people diagnosed with schizophrenia has been associated with living longer. In a study using Finnish nationwide databases (Taipale et al., 2020), of the people with schizophrenia who were not dispensed medication, 46.2% were dead within 20 years, compared to 25.7% of the group who were dispensed any antipsychotic drug at any time.

REFERENCES

Andreason, N. C., Carpenter, W. T., Kane, J. M., Lasser, R. A., Marder, R. R., & Weinberger, D. R. (2005). Remission in schizophrenia: Proposed criteria and rationale for consensus. *American Journal of Psychiatry* 162:441–449.

Ascher-Svanum, H., Faries, D. E., Zhu, B., Ernst, F. R., Swartz, M. S., & Swanson, J. W. (2006). Medication adherence and long-term functional outcomes in the treatment of schizophrenia in usual care. *Journal of Clinical Psychiatry* 67(3):453–460.

Carbon, M., & Correll, C. U. (2014). Clinical predictors of therapeutic response to antipsychotics in schizophrenia. *Dialogues in Clinical Neuroscience* 16(4):505–524.

Caseiro, O., Perez-Iglesias, R., Mata, I., Martinez-Garcia, O., Pelayo-Teran, J. M., Taberas-Seisdedos, R., Ortiz-Garcia de la Foz, V., Vazquez-Barquero, J. L., & Crespo-Facorro, B. (2012). Predicting relapse after a first episode of non-affective psychosis: A three-year follow-up study. *Journal of Psychiatric Research* 46:1099–1105.

Karow, A., Naber, D., Lambert, M., & Moritz, S. (2012). Remission as perceived by people with schizophrenia, family members and psychiatrists. *European Psychiatry* 6:426–431.

Kay, S. R., Fiszbein, A., & Opler, L. A. (1987). The Positive and Negative Syndrome Scale for Schizophrenia (PANSS). *Schizophrenia Bulletin* 13(2):261–276.

Lambert, M., Karow, A., Leucht, S., Schimmelmann, B. G., & Naber, D. (2010). Remission in schizophrenia: Validity, frequency, predictors, and patient's perspective 5 years later. *Dialogues in Clinical Neuroscience* 12(3):393–407.

Lambert, M., Naber, D., Schacht, A., Wagner, T., Hundemer, H. P., Karow, A., . . . & Dittman, R. W. (2008). Rates and predictors of remission and recovery during 3 years in 392 never-treated patients with schizophrenia. *Acta Psychiatrica Scandanavica* 118:220–229.

Lambert, M., Schimmelmann, B. G., Naber, D., Schacht, A., Karow, A., Waner, T., & Czekalla, J. (2006). Prediction of remission as a combination of symptomatic and functional remission and adequate subjective well-being in 2960 patients with schizophrenia. *Journal of Clinical Psychiatry* 67(11):1690–1697.

Leucht, S., Tardy, M., Komossa, K., Heres, S., Kissling, W., Salanti, G., & Davis, J. M. (2012). Antipsychotic drugs versus placebo for relapse prevention in schizophrenia: A systemic review and meta-analysis. *Lancet* 379 (9831):2063–2071.

Novick, D., Haro, J. M., Suarez, D., Perez, V., Dittmann, R. W., & Hadda, P. M. (2010). Predictors and clinical consequences of non-adherence with antipsychotic medication in the outpatient treatment of schizophrenia. *Psychiatry Research* 176:109–113.

Olfson, M., Mechanic, D., Hansell, S., Boyer, C. S., Walkup, J., & Weiden, P. J. (2000). Predicting medication noncompliance after hospital discharge among patients with schizophrenia. *Psychiatric Services* 51(2):216–222.

Overall, J. E., & Gorham, D. R. (1962). The Brief Psychiatric Rating Scale. *Psychological Reports* 10(3):799–812.

Taipale, H., Tanskanen, A., Mehtala, J., Vattulainen, P., Correll, C. U., & Tiihonen, J. (2020). 20-year follow-up study of physical morbidity and mortality in relationship to antipsychotic treatment in a nationwide cohort of 62,250 patients with schizophrenia (FIN20). *World Psychiatry* 19(1):61–68.

Van Dee, V., Schnack, H. G., & Cahn, W. (2023). Systematic review and meta-analysis on predictors of prognosis in patients with schizophrenia spectrum disorders: An overview of current evidence and a call for prospective research and open access to datasets. *Schizophrenia Research* 254:133–142.

Ventura, J., Subotnik, K. L., Guzik, L. H., Hellemann, G. S., Gitlin, M. J., Wood, R. C., & Nuechterlein, K. H. (2011). Remission and recovery during the first outpatient year of the early course of schizophrenia. *Schizophrenia Research* 132(1):18–23.

3.5 CASE F: BORN OF BRITISH ROYALTY

3.5.1 Case

Mr. F. was a man in his early 30s when he was sent to a state psychiatric hospital directly from prison upon completion of his sentence.

History

Mr. F.'s first contact with psychiatry was in prison. Corrections officers charged him with numerous disciplinary violations, such as property destruction and refusing direct orders, and also noticed that he refused to speak with his mother when she visited. They referred him to mental health services. When initially interviewed by a social worker, she noted that Mr. F. was withdrawn and responded to internal stimuli. Soon thereafter, a psychiatrist concluded that he was psychotic and in need of involuntary hospital treatment.

Course of treatment

Early on, the new patient sat off in a corner of his ward alone. His mother came to visit regularly, but, to her dismay, he insisted she was not his mother and his name was not Mr. F. When asked for his thoughts about discharge, he insisted that he should be allowed to return to Great Britain to be reunited with his real family, the royal family. Though he was offered a number of antipsychotic drugs, he refused all.

His psychiatrist obtained an order for treatment over objection with long-acting intramuscular haloperidol. With this treatment he became less isolated in that he kept abreast of US and world news and occasionally chose to leave his ward with other patients and a staff member escort. After his court order expired, he accepted injections willingly and agreed to remain in the hospital as a voluntary patient. Still, he usually sat alone in his favorite corner, did not speak spontaneously to anyone, and insisted he was a member of the House of Windsor.

Mr. F. refused a trial of clozapine but accepted olanzapine. With this change he took better care with his personal appearance and began to initiate contact with other people. Gradually, he became involved in ward activities to the point that he became a leader, speaking up for the group in community meetings.

On interview, he was neat, cleanly shaven, alert, attentive, and able to express himself clearly. In discussions with his doctor, he took an active interest in psychiatric diagnosis and treatments. Mr. F. recognized that he had changed and that medication had helped him do so. The only indication he was ill was that he still insisted he was a British royal and that the woman who, in reality, was his mother, was not.

His immediate goal was to obtain a job within the hospital. Longer-term goals were to leave the hospital, live in a community residence in a nice neighborhood with tree-lined streets, and eventually get a job as an apprentice plumber. He was not interested in discharge anytime soon.

Mr. F. secured and performed well in a custodial job in a patient work program off his ward. He always accepted prescribed medication and wanted to continue doing so after discharge. With time, his conviction that he was born into royalty and must be discharged to the United Kingdom disappeared, but he continued to maintain that his mother was not his mother. While this was a source of sorrow to his mother, it was not a reason to continue hospitalization.

His ward social worker presented him with options for supportive housing. While he refused an offer of a quick move to transitional housing in the hospital's on-grounds residence, he agreed to wait and apply for an independent scatter-site apartment.

3.5.2 Pay for patient workers

Working gave Mr. F. a sense of accomplishment and money to save. The 1973 *Souder v. Brennan* federal court ruling required that patient workers in institutions for the mentally ill and mentally retarded be paid in accordance with the minimum wage. The ruling was contrary to widely accepted practices of the time (Safier, 1976).

REFERENCES

Safier, D. (1976). Patient work under fair labor standards: The issue in perspective. *Psychiatric Services* 27(2):89–92.
Souder v. Brennan. 367 F. Supp. 808 (D.D.C. 1973).

3.6 HOW DO ANTIPSYCHOTIC DRUGS COMPARE?

3.6.1 Efficacy

Guidelines published by the American Psychiatric Association (APA) state that there is no definitive evidence that one antipsychotic drug will have consistently superior efficacy compared with another, with the possible exception of clozapine (American Psychiatric Association, 2021).

Overall, evidence for greater effectiveness of any antipsychotic besides clozapine and long-acting injectables (LAIs) is not conclusive, although there may be a modest advantage for some, but not all, second-generation agents compared to first-generation agents (Miyamoto & Fleischhaker, 2012). A meta-analysis (Leucht et al., 2023) concluded that olanzapine is more efficacious than several other first- and second-generation drugs although olanzapine's advantage ranged from very small when compared to risperidone, to small to medium when compared to ziprasidone.

3.6.2 LAIs and clozapine for preventing relapse

The APA Guidelines suggests use of a depot or long-acting injectable antipsychotic (LAI) if patients prefer this or have a history of poor or uncertain adherence (American Psychiatric Association, 2021), which many patients do. LAIs perform better than oral drugs in preventing relapse due to improved adherence. Real-world naturalistic studies are best suited to detecting this advantage (Bossie, 2015).

An example of one such study used the database of the public healthcare provider in Hong Kong (Wei et al., 2022). Investigators compared times when individuals with schizophrenia were prescribed any oral antipsychotic, including clozapine but excluding a LAI, to times when the same person was prescribed only a LAI. Compared to oral drugs, depot preparations were associated with a 47% lower rate of hospitalizations for schizophrenia and a 44% decrease in suicide attempts. Findings were similar for patients with comorbid substance abuse and people older than 65.

Using a Swedish nationwide database and similar methods, investigators (Tiihonen et al., 2017) compared times when individuals with schizophrenia were prescribed a particular drug compared to times when the same person was not. The risk of rehospitalization was 22% lower during use of a LAI compared to use of an oral formulation of the same drug. Compared to when patients were taking the most commonly used drug, olanzapine, the lowest risk of death, hospitalization, drug discontinuation, or switch occurred when patients were on clozapine. The second lowest risk was for all LAIs.

3.6.3 Side effects

Antipsychotic drugs differ greatly in their side-effect profiles. Common adverse effects of newer or second-generation antipsychotics (e.g., olanzapine, risperidone, and clozapine) are weight gain, which can be marked, as well as glucose and lipid dysregulation and elevated prolactin levels. In men, elevated prolactin is manifested as sexual dysfunction. Sedation and decreased blood pressure are also possible (Miyamoto & Fleischhaker, 2012).

Older, first-generation drugs can be either high-potency (i.e., producing more effect per milligram) or low-potency. Common adverse effects of high-potency drugs (e.g., haloperidol and fluphenazine) are extrapyramidal symptoms (EPS), which include tremor, muscle stiffness, acute muscle spasm or dystonia, and restlessness or akathisia. EPS are reversible with decreased dosing, change in antipsychotic agent, or addition of an adjuvant agent (e.g., benztropine) (Miyamoto & Fleischhaker, 2012). Low-potency agents such as chlorpromazine are less likely to cause EPS but more likely to cause sedation, postural hypotension, and anticholinergic effects, such as dry mouth and constipation (Schatzberg & DeBattista, 2015).

Tardive dyskinesia (TD) is possible with the use of all antipsychotic drugs. It is more concerning than EPS because it is potentially irreversible (Miyamoto & Fleischhaker, 2012). TD is usually manifested by involuntary, repetitive movements mostly in the mouth, lips, tongue, and cheeks, but also in other parts of the face, extremities, and torso (Correll et al., 2017). Patients age 55 and older are more susceptible (Woerner et al., 1998).

A review of many studies (Carbon et al., 2018), of which more than 80% used standardized screening tools, estimated that the rate of new-onset TD per year of treatment is 6.5% for first-generation drugs and 2.6% for second-generation drugs. In studies that used only clinical reporting, which would detect less subtle, more easily recognized abnormal movements, the incidence was 3.8% per year of treatment for first-generation and 0.9% for second-generation drugs. Reports of severe cases were rare. The risk to develop TD is cumulative, at least during the first 5 years of treatment, so a typical patient's lifetime risk is much higher than their annual risk.

The prevalence of TD in people with schizophrenia or similar disorders on antipsychotics varies widely, but one group (Carbon et al., 2017) estimated an average prevalence of 25% as detected by rating scales.

REFERENCES

American Psychiatric Association. (2021). Pharmacotherapy. In *Practice Guideline for the Treatment of Patients with Schizophrenia*, 3rd ed. Eds. G. A. Keeper et al., pp. 33–118. Washington, DC: American Psychiatric Publishing.

Bossie, C. A., Alphs, L. D., & Correll, C. U. (2015). Long-acting injectable versus daily oral antipsychotic treatment trials in schizophrenia: Pragmatic versus explanatory study designs. *International Clinical Psychopharmacology* 30(5):272–281.

Carbon, M., Kane, J. M., Leucht, S., & Correll, C. U. (2018). Tardive dyskinesia risk with first- and second-generation antipsychotics in comparative randomized controlled trials: A meta-analysis. *World Psychiatry* 173(3):330–340.

Carbon, M., Hsieh, C-H., Kane, J. M., & Correll, C. U. (2017). Tardive dyskinesia prevalence in the period of second-generation antipsychotic use: A meta-analysis. *Journal of Clinical Psychiatry* 78(3):330–340.

Correll, C. C., Kane, J. M., & Citrome, L. J. (2017). Epidemiology, prevention and assessment of tardive dyskinesia and advances in treatment. *Journal of Clinical Psychiatry* 78(8):1136–1147.

Leucht, S., Schneider-Thoma, J., Burschinski, A., Peter, N., Wang, D., Dong, S., . . ., & Davis, J. M. (2023). Long-term efficacy of antipsychotic drugs in initially acutely ill adults with schizophrenia: Systematic review and network meta-analysis. *World Psychiatry* 22(2):315–324.

Miyamoto, S., & Fleischhaker, W. W. (2012). Pharmacologic treatment of schizophrenia. In *Clinical Manual for Treatment of Schizophrenia*. Eds. J. Lauriello & S. Pallani, pp. 291–340. Washington, DC: American Psychiatric Publishing.

Schatzberg, A. F., & DeBattista, C. (2015). *Manual of Clinical Psychopharmacology*, 8th ed. Washington, DC: American Psychiatric Publishing.

Tiihonen, J., Mittendorfer-Rutz, E., Majak, M., Mehtala, J., Hoti, F., Jedenius, E., . . . & Taipale, H. (2017). Real-world effectiveness of antipsychotic treatments in a nationwide cohort of 29,823 patients with schizophrenia. *JAMA Psychiatry* 74(7):686–693.

Wei, Y., Yan, V. K. C., Kang, W., Wong, I. C. K., Castle, D. J., Goa, L., . . . & Chan, E. W. (2022). Association of long-acting injectable antipsychotics and oral antipsychotics with disease relapse, health care use, and adverse effects among people with schizophrenia, *JAMA Network Open* 5(7):e2224163. doi: 10.1001/jamanetworkopen.2022.24163. PMID: 35900760; PMCID: PMC9335136.

Woerner, M. G., Alvir, J. M., Saltz, B. L., Lieberman, J. A., & Kane, J. M. (1998). Prospective study of tardive dyskinesia in the elderly: Rates and risk factors. *American Journal of Psychiatry* 155(11):1521–1528.

3.7 INDIVIDUALIZED PRESCRIBING

The goals of prescribing are efficacy and tolerability, or, in other words, to improve symptoms enough to maximize a patient's functioning and minimize distress, including the distress of adverse effects. Eliminating all symptoms is often not possible. Eliminating all adverse effects may be difficult. When a patient cannot tolerate an effective dose of one agent, a drug with different adverse effects may show better results.

Two to four weeks may be needed for some initial drug response and additional time for a full response. Patients are more likely to tolerate a slow dose escalation than a rapid one (American Psychiatric Association, 2021).

Choice and dosing depend on the patient's medical conditions. For example, preexisting obesity and diabetes should be a consideration in choosing drugs that are more likely to exacerbate these conditions. Choice and dosing also depend on patient characteristics and preferences. Older adults may be more sensitive to adverse effects. Dosing also depends on chronicity, because first-episode patients may require less medication (American Psychiatric Association, 2021). Paranoid patients can be especially sensitive to adverse effects and take them as evidence of the malign nature of medication and the ill intent of the doctor. For some patients, sedation, a common side effect, can be welcome.

When prescribing for a person who has used antipsychotics in the past, history and the patient's attitude to past treatments are guides. American Psychiatric Association (APA) Practice guideline suggests that patients whose symptoms have improved with a particular antipsychotic medication in the past be treated with the same medication going forward (American Psychiatric Association, 2021). The drug that the patient is willing to take and finds helpful has a clear advantage.

In continuing an antipsychotic, follow target symptoms, patient functioning, distress, and adverse effects. Consider patient report and the reports from treatment team members and family, if possible. Clinicians need to understand what the patient reports and if it is related to medication. Patients often use idiosyncratic language and may attribute any uncomfortable feeling, including symptoms of psychotic illness, to medication.

REFERENCE

American Psychiatric Association. (2021). Pharmacotherapy. In *Practice Guideline for the Treatment of Patients with Schizophrenia*, 3rd ed. Eds. G. A. Keepers et al., pp. 33–118. Washington, DC: American Psychiatric Press.

4

SCHIZOPHRENIA OR SOMETHING ELSE?

As patients reveal themselves and more history becomes available, state hospitals can undertake a diagnostic reassessment and offer more effective, appropriate treatment. This chapter offers guidance on how to distinguish schizophrenia from other disorders and reviews the association of auditory hallucinations and trauma. Three cases illustrate diagnostic distinctions.

4.1 CASE G: WHAT'S HAPPENING WITH ME?

4.1.1 Case

Mr. G. was a young African-American man who was arrested and charged with a misdemeanor. After he was found not fit to stand trial, his charges were dropped and he was transferred from jail to a state hospital.

Interview

Mr. G. had an old, well-healed scar alongside a new, superficial, still healing laceration on his wrist. Immediately upon sitting for his admission interview he asked for food. After his psychiatrist, Dr. B., handed him a sandwich, the young man eagerly gobbled it down. Mr. G. was nearly inaudible, so Dr. B. asked him to pull his chair a little closer in order to hear him better. Mr. G. complied without hesitation. Both his speech and his movements were excruciatingly slow. He yawned and looked at the floor, expressionless, and repeatedly asked to rest. When asked about his mood, he asked to rest. He said he did not experience hallucinations, but also that he didn't like being around a lot of people because they could hurt him. He denied current suicidal ideas. Then, for a second, he made contact. He lifted his head and asked, "What's happening with me?"

History

Mr. G.'s mother reported to her son's treatment team that he had lost interest in life years earlier. He had friends and dated in high school but, midway through, dropped out and spent his time just hanging out at home. Briefly, he took a job bagging groceries but he soon returned to lying around and sleeping all day. He was afraid of crowds, spoke very softly, and had no friends and no romantic interests. His mother did not see evidence he was using illicit drugs or drinking alcohol.

Her son had previous psychiatric assessments on two occasions. After a suicide attempt by cutting his wrist, he was hospitalized and treated with divalproex and methylphenidate. On another occasion, he had an emergency room evaluation, a "see and release," when psychiatrists evaluated and then released him. After both assessments he was scheduled for ongoing treatment at an outpatient clinic, but he did not appear.

In the month before his arrest, Mr. G.'s condition deteriorated. His mother said he was spending most of his time in a daze, watching television, avoiding others, and rarely speaking, but then he started to claim he was appearing on the television and that people were talking about him. As the month progressed, his behavior became stranger and more concerning: he stopped bathing and changing his clothes, destroyed his television, and allegedly committed a crime.

Sitting in a jail cell for the first time ever, he superficially cut his wrist. A psychiatrist employed by the jail noted paranoia, depressed mood, poverty of thought, and threatening and assaultive gestures. The psychiatrist diagnosed schizophrenia and started olanzapine.

When Mr. G. appeared in court, his mother advocated for psychiatric treatment instead of a jail sentence.

Course of treatment

Mr. G. was continued on the medication he was prescribed in jail, olanzapine 15 mg. One quiet afternoon, Dr. B., a man old enough to be his grandfather, was sitting alone in a conference room engrossed in patient records when Mr. G. slipped in and sat down. He implored, "What's happening to me? Am I gonna be alright?" He said he felt very sad, lost, alone, and trapped and didn't know what to do. He feared nothing would change, that he was going to mess up. His psychiatrist spoke to him softly and empathically.

At that point, Dr. B. came to understand that his patient was depressed. He prescribed paroxetine in addition to olanzapine. In the next week, instead of sleeping in the dayroom, Mr. G. started attending therapeutic groups. There he was attentive but asked nothing, and, if addressed, gave a barely audible reply and looked down. He never smiled. In another week, he played cards with other patients. When greeted, he looked up and nodded. He was eager to take medication.

In his fourth week, he had more to say and said it more loudly, but offered only short replies including, "I don't know." He looked down, undecided, and then volunteered that he felt better than he had in a long time.

In the following weeks, Mr. G. initiated entirely audible conversations with ward staff and joked and chatted with other patients. He spoke spontaneously and in long sentences, looked his psychiatrist directly in the eye, smiled, and said hello. In groups, he read psychoeducational material loud enough for all to hear, listened intently, and laughed out loud, but did not volunteer comments. In meetings with his treatment team, he expressed hope for his future and revealed plans to further his formal education. He said he felt better, no longer sad, but wanted to stay in the hospital until he felt better still.

By the eighth week, Mr. G. and his mother met with his psychiatrist and social worker to plan his discharge. "I'm feeling good," he said. "I'm getting old and ready to move on. I want a nice quiet place to live." He was certain that he would continue to take his medication.

4.2 IS IT AN AFFECTIVE DISORDER?

4.2.1 Variability of psychiatric diagnoses

Psychiatric diagnoses made by different clinicians or at different times by the same clinician are often inconsistent. This can be due to the evolution of a patient's illness over time (e.g., from major depressive disorder to bipolar disorder), to the availability of more information, or to various clinicians' points of view. Diagnoses can vary between treatment settings, with the patient's race, and with use of structured versus clinical interviews.

A large study over the course of 4 years found that the main variable influencing diagnostic stability was the setting in which patients were assessed (Baca-Garcia et al., 2007). Of patients who were assessed at least 10 times, those who were assessed in hospitals compared to emergency rooms were more likely to receive the same diagnosis for at least 75% of evaluations.

A review of research conducted over 24 years (Schwartz & Blankenship, 2014) concluded that African Americans are three to five times more likely to be diagnosed with schizophrenia than are White Americans, with similar results for Hispanic-Americans. One particular study of 2,311 patients admitted to a state hospital in Indiana over the course of 8 years determined that Black patients were four times more likely than White patients to be diagnosed with schizophrenia (Barnes, 2004).

When diagnoses are obtained via structured interviews, they are more consistent. Researchers working in an outpatient psychiatric rehabilitation facility (Kotwicki & Harvey, 2013) compared admission diagnoses made by referring clinicians to discharge diagnoses made by treating clinicians after a facility stay averaging 13 weeks. Discharge diagnosis differed from admission diagnosis in 74% of 313 cases. When admission diagnoses were obtained with structured interviews, change rates were much lower, 4% or 11%, depending on the structured interview used. Researchers also noted if admission diagnoses were confirmed by structured interviews. Forty to 65% of bipolar disorder and major depression admission diagnoses were confirmed. Admission diagnoses of bipolar disorder were often changed to major depression, and diagnoses of major depression were often changed to bipolar depression. Confirmation of schizoaffective referral diagnoses was very low, 10–11%.

4.2.2 Affective disorders versus schizophrenia

Depression with psychotic symptoms

Returning to our case study from the preceding chapter, the psychiatrist working at the jail where he was incarcerated examined Mr. G. and noted depressed mood, a psychotic symptom (paranoia) and a negative symptom (poverty of thought). The doctor diagnosed schizophrenia. But psychotic symptoms are not specific to schizophrenia, and negative symptoms can be indistinguishable from symptoms of depression. For clinicians examining individual patients, *anhedonia*, the decreased ability to experience pleasure, is not different from the markedly diminished interest or pleasure in regular activities seen in major depressive disorder. *Avolition*, a decrease in motivated, self-initiated purposeful activities, is not different from Mr. G.'s psychomotor retardation. Mr. G. also showed the negative symptom, *alogia*, or diminished speech output, which could be described as poverty of thought. This phenomena could be attributed to his fatigue or loss of energy—a depressive symptom. It is indistinguishable from another depressive symptom, *diminished ability to think* (American Psychiatric Association, 2022a, 2022b).

To make diagnosis more difficult, some individuals have both schizophrenia and depression. In other words, "mood symptoms and full mood episodes are common in schizophrenia and may be concurrent with active-phase symptomatology" (American Psychiatric Association, 2022a, p.115). Suicidal ideation and attempts occur both in people with major depressive disorder and in people with schizophrenia. About 20% of people with schizophrenia attempt suicide and 5–6% die by suicide. Suicidal behavior may be linked to command hallucinations but also to depressive symptoms (American Psychiatric Association, 2022a). In deciding if a person with schizophrenia is also depressed, the presence of low mood, suicidal ideas, and pessimism point to depression, but alogia and blunted affect are more specific to schizophrenia (Krynicki et al., 2018).

Bipolar disorder

People with schizophrenia can be angry, agitated, or grandiose. Mania is distinguished by a persistent change. It requires a distinct period of abnormally and persistently elevated or irritable mood along with persistently increased activity or energy most of the day, nearly every day, for a week (American Psychiatric Association, 2022b). Chapter 2.3 presents a good example of a man with mania.

Schizoaffective disorder

Because Mr. G. had both affective and psychotic symptoms some clinicians would diagnose schizoaffective disorder. But making this choice without carefully considering other options, options with distinct prognoses and treatments, can lead to suboptimal care.

Schizoaffective disorder is a popular diagnosis among clinicians but controversial. Clinicians rarely agree on its diagnosis, as Kotwicki and Harvey (2013) found. Some have questioned its validity as separate from psychotic mood disorder and suggest it should be eliminated from the diagnostic nomenclature (Lake & Hurwitz, 2007).

Schizoaffective disorder requires a review of the duration of the patient's illness. Symptoms of a mood disorder must be present for most of the duration, while delusions or hallucinations are present for 2 weeks or more in the absence of a major mood episode. Mr. G.'s illness did not meet these criteria because he had mood symptoms throughout the course of his illness (American Psychiatric Association, 2022a).

REFERENCES

American Psychiatric Association. (2022a). Schizophrenia spectrum and other psychotic disorders. In *Diagnostic and Statistical Manual of Mental Disorders*, 5th ed., text revision, pp. 101–136. Washington, DC: American Psychiatric Association.

American Psychiatric Association. (2022b). Bipolar and related disorders. In *Diagnostic and Statistical Manual of Mental Disorders*, 5th ed., text revision, pp. 139–175. Washington, DC: American Psychiatric Association.

Baca-Garcia, E., Perez-Rodriguez, M. M., Basurte-Villamor, I., Fernandez del Moreal, F., Jimenez-Arriero, M. A. Gonzalez de Rivera, J. L., . . . & Oquendo, M. A. (2007). Diagnostic stability of psychiatric disorders in clinical practice. *British Journal of Psychiatry* 190:210–216.

Barnes, A. (2004). Race, schizophrenia, and admission to state psychiatric hospitals. *Administration and Policy in Mental Health* (3):241–252.

Kotwicki, R., & Harvey, P. D. (2013). Systematic study of structured diagnostic procedures in outpatient psychiatric rehabilitation: A three-year, three-cohort study of the stability of psychiatric diagnoses. *Innovations in Clinical Neuroscience* 10(5-6):14–19.

Krynicki, C. R., Uptegrove, R., Deakin, J. F. W., & Barnes, T. R. E. (2018). The relationship between negative symptoms and depression in schizophrenia: A systematic review. *Acta Psychiatrica Scandanavica* 137(5):380–390.

Lake, C. R., & Hurwitz, N. (2007). Schizoaffective disorder merges schizophrenia and bipolar disorders as one disease: There is no schizoaffective disorder. *Current Opinion in Psychiatry* 20(4):365–379.

Schwartz, R. C., & Blankenship, D. M. (2014). Racial disparities in psychotic disorder diagnosis: A review of empirical literature. *World Journal of Psychiatry* 4(4):133–140.

4.3 CASE H: THE MAN WHO WANTED AMBIEN

4.3.1 Case

Mr. H. was a man in his late 60s who was transferred to a state hospital from a community hospital with a diagnosis of schizoaffective disorder and history of a back injury.

Interview

On admission Mr. H.'s responses were logical, direct, and unelaborated. His first and most vociferous complaint was back pain. Just as insistently he claimed that the only treatment that had ever alleviated his pain was zolpidem. His mood was down, his sleep and appetite poor. In his future, he wanted to get out of the hospital, stay out of places like it, and find a small apartment. He said that no, he had never in his life experienced auditory hallucinations.

He reported a series of admissions to a state hospital as a teenager and young adult due to problems getting along with his mother. After each hospital discharge he returned to his mother's apartment. Following his final state hospitalization he worked steadily for more than 20 years for an hourly wage and then intermittently for another few years. Mr. H. lived with his mother in her apartment until she died, and he remained there, alone, after her death. A fire forced him to leave 3 years before his current state hospital stay.

His zolpidem use began because pain from a back injury kept him awake at night. When he could not obtain it by prescription, he bought it on the street. One day when he was living in a shelter, he took 30 or 40 mg, then blacked out and woke up in the emergency room.

History

Review of records revealed that Mr. H. was admitted to state psychiatric hospitals several times from the late 1950s, when he was a teenager, to the late 1960s. His first and all subsequent admissions were due to his mother's complaints of behavior problems, which in later years included substance abuse. During all his hospital stays he did not show evidence of psychosis.

About 50 years after his last state hospital discharge he was sent to a community hospital emergency room from a shelter because he had been seen mostly naked, wandering aimlessly, and trying to eat nonedible objects such as a sock. In the emergency room, he was described as inattentive, with loose associations and bizarre delusions (e.g., that he was in a spaceship). On admission, ward clinicians wrote that he remained bizarre and isolated, and complained of insomnia. They noted a history of prior state hospital treatment and of fire-setting, both of which contributed to the decision to transfer him to a state hospital for longer-term care.

Course of treatment

Mr. H. was initially continued on the medication regimen he was taking at the referring hospital, which was haloperidol decanoate 100 mg intramuscularly every month, duloxetine 60 mg daily, and naproxen for chronic pain. Soon after admission he lay on the floor whenever he got a chance and complained of back pain, thus frustrating ward attendants who repeatedly urged him to get up and join treatment groups or sit with other patients. After a review of his distant history and of later treatment records, Mr. H. was taken off antipsychotic medication.

Second interview

Some weeks later he was more spontaneous and able to provide more information. Back pain was still his most urgent complaint. In addition, he said his mood was sad, his sleep poor, his energy level low, and his enjoyment of food under par. He wanted to die but dismissed ideas of killing himself in the hospital, where he saw no options to do so.

Mr. H. filled in more of his history. After his last 1960s state hospital discharge he was treated inconsistently with antidepressants as an outpatient but was not hospitalized until 3 years before his current hospital stay. That admission occurred after a fire destroyed his apartment, a fire he set, accidentally, by smoking in bed. "My whole life was in that place," he said mournfully. When asked how he paid the rent, he said that he did not, that at the time of the fire he was almost 2 years behind. "It was crack," he said, "I used to do this thing called crack."

After hospital discharge he resided in various shelters and adult homes and, once, in another hospital. He said that he had to move when he did not meet the expectations of adult homes. For example, he was forced out of one when staff found cigarettes butts in his dresser drawer. Living in such places was like being a sheep in a pack, he said, so he preferred his own place.

Course of treatment

Duloxetine was increased to 90 mg daily, then stopped for lack of efficacy. Citalopram was started for depression, and his pain was treated more aggressively. Mr. H. gradually spent less time complaining of pain and lying on the floor. While he remained a loner, he would attend groups with much encouragement or sit in the dayroom. He was eventually discharged but not to his own place.

4.3.2 Comment

Like Mr. G., Mr. H. received a diagnostic reassessment. Mr. H.'s reassessment was based on access to old hospital records but was also based on ward observation and interviews. Referring psychiatrists diagnosed both men with chronic psychotic disorders, schizophrenia for Mr. H. and schizoaffective illness for Mr. G. Both cases illustrate the variety of diagnoses associated with psychotic symptoms and the need to distinguish the negative symptoms of chronic psychotic illness from symptoms of depression.

4.4 IS IT SUBSTANCE-INDUCED DELIRIUM?

Mr. H. was taken off antipsychotics because his symptoms in the emergency room seemed likely due to abuse of a substance (i.e., zolpidem), and his past history did not show evidence of psychotic illness. Zolpidem has a reputation for low abuse potential, but abuse, dependence, and withdrawal have been reported in the United States and abroad (Hajak et al., 2003; Madrak & Rosenberg, 2021; Victorri-Vigneau et al, 2007). Delirium and psychosis with zolpidem use have also been reported (Markowitz & Brewerton, 1996; Tsai et al., 2003).

Zolpidem is an unusual offender, but delirium can be caused by intoxication with many substances: alcohol, cannabis, phencyclidine and other hallucinogens, inhalants, opioids, stimulants, cocaine, sedative/hypnotics, and other drugs. In addition, it can be caused by substance withdrawal, medications, toxins, or medical illnesses (American Psychiatric Association, 2022a).

When seen in the emergency room, Mr. H. met criteria for substance-intoxication delirium. He had a disturbance in consciousness with inability to focus attention. He had a perceptual disturbance in that he believed he was in a spaceship. Critically, Mr. H.'s disturbance developed over hours to days.

Delirium or another substance-induced disorder are distinguished from schizophrenia or schizoaffective disorder by the presence of one of the above etiological factors and the truncated time course of the disturbance (American Psychiatric Association, 2022a). No previous history of psychotic illness is another indication, as is clearing without use of antipsychotic drugs.

Patients may have both conditions, schizophrenia or another chronic psychotic illness, and delirium. Rates of comorbidity for substance-related disorders and schizophrenia are high (American Psychiatric Association, 2022b), as they are with bipolar disorder (American Psychiatric Association, 2022c) (see Chapter 8.4 for an example). Seriously mentally ill people can also have medical problems that can cause delirium. They might also have a psychotic chronic illness with exacerbations due to other factors (e.g., nonadherence).

To make the differential diagnosis, look for an etiologic factor, perform urine toxicology screens, and look for confusion and a presentation atypical for that patient. Patients with recurrent psychotic episodes have similar delusions across episodes (Grunfield et al., 2024).

REFERENCES

American Psychiatric Association. (2022a). Neurocognitive disorders. In *Diagnostic and Statistical Manual of Mental Disorders*, 5th ed., text revision, pp. 667–732. Washington, DC: American Psychiatric Association.

American Psychiatric Association. (2022b). Schizophrenia spectrum and other psychotic disorders. In *Diagnostic and Statistical Manual of Mental Disorders*, 5th ed., text revision, pp. 101–136. Washington, DC: American Psychiatric Association.

American Psychiatric Association. (2022c). Bipolar and related disorders. In *Diagnostic and Statistical Manual of Mental Disorders*, 5th ed., text revision, pp. 139–175. Washington, DC: American Psychiatric Association.

Grunfield, G., Lemonde, A.-C., Gold, I., Paquin, V., Iyer, S. N., Lepage, M., . . . & Shah, J. L. (2024). Consistency of delusion themes across first and subsequent episodes of psychosis. *JAMA Psychiatry* 81(10):1039–1046.

Hajak, G., Muller, W. E., Wittchen, H. U., Pittrow, D., & Kirch, W. (2003). Abuse and dependence potential for the non-benzodiazepine hypnotics zolpidem and zopiclone: A review of case reports and epidemiological data. *Addiction* 98(10):1371–1378.

Madrak, L. N., & Rosenberg, M. (2021). Zolpidem abuse. *American Journal of Psychiatry* 158:1330–1331.

Markowitz, J. S., & Brewerton, T. D. (1996). Zolpidem-induced psychosis. *Annals of Clinical Psychiatry* 8(2):89–91.

Tsai, M. J., Huang, Y. B., & Wu, P. C. (2003). A novel clinical pattern of visual hallucination after zolpidem use. *Journal of Toxicology and Clinical Toxicology* 41(6):869–872.

Victorri-Vigneau, C., Dailly, E., Veyrac, G., & Jolliet, P. (2007). Evidence of zolpidem abuse and dependence: Results of the French Centre for Evaluation and Information on Pharmacodependence (CEIP) network survey. *British Journal of Clinical Pharmacology* 64(2): 198–209.

4.5 CASE I: TRAVELING BETWEEN TIME ZONES

4.5.1 Case

Mr. I. was a man in his late 40s who was admitted to a state psychiatric hospital after he was charged with throwing around and destroying merchandise in small convenience store—a misdemeanor—and found not fit to stand trial. While in jail, he was offered and accepted haloperidol 5 mg twice daily and benztropine 1 mg twice daily.

Interview

On admission, Mr. I. was a polite and attentive man who readily answered all questions coherently and with feeling. He denied all current symptoms, including hallucinations, but when pressed, he waffled, and then admitted to a strange belief: that some people could move from one time zone to another. He did not understand why he was currently in a hospital, but he knew what he wanted for his future. His wish was to find a place to live and a job, but he feared he could not because his birth certificate and Social Security card had been lost.

Mr. I. said he had been living with and caring for his frail grandfather, supported by the older man's Social Security benefits. When the elderly man died, Mr. I. was sad, all alone, and slept poorly but for 2 months made efforts to obtain income and stay in his apartment. When his efforts failed and he lost his apartment, he stayed a few days with friends here, a few days with friends somewhere else, and then landed on the streets. Four days after he began walking the streets, he was arrested.

The new patient could not logically explain why he destroyed property in the small store, only that he thought the place was his home. With embarrassment and regret he related that he had drank a few beers and was feeling a little depressed, a little confused, and was imagining things, foolish things such as that he was in a different time zone. He denied that he was hearing voices at the time. Two days after his arrest, he was all over it.

His only previous contact with psychiatry occurred several years earlier, when his mother died. Just as when his grandfather died, he became very upset and wandered the streets for a few days, moving between time zones and talking to himself, but not experiencing hallucinations. After he was taken to a hospital and given medication, he calmed down and was soon released. Within a few days he recovered and was able to return to supporting himself and caring for his grandfather. Mr. I. said the idea of travel between time zones was embarrassing and nonsensical, but added that he was affected in this way because he had bickered with his stepfather.

Mr. I. was very close to his grandfather because as a child he often lived with him, though he also spent time with his mother and stepfather. He initially denied substance abuse, then admitted to smoking marijuana each day for about a year before admission.

History

Fitness examiners obtained the same history, except that Mr. I. told them that voices had told him to enter the store, voices which at the time seemed real, but which, in retrospect, he believed were his own thoughts. They noted that he was socially isolated and demonstrated an inappropriate affect when discussing his crime. They diagnosed brief psychotic disorder, but also suggested that schizophrenia was another possibility.

Course of treatment

Because the newly admitted patient reported no psychotic symptoms and his episode occurred while he was smoking marijuana, his psychiatrist discontinued haloperidol and benztropine. After a few days, he told his psychiatrist he felt no different. The doctor noted that he kept to himself on the ward.

Nine days after his admission, he became tearful after a telephone call with a family member, then approached a nurse and complained of sadness and hearing voices. Mr. I. confessed that he had feared he would remain in the hospital for years and years if he revealed that he had been experiencing auditory hallucinations from when he was in sixth grade, almost continuously. The voices distracted him when he worked. They often spoke gibberish, but at times were clearly deprecating and at other times positive and supportive. He never believed they were his own thoughts, but believed they came from inside his brain. With antipsychotic treatment they had stopped, but with discontinuation they resumed. When asked about what happened in the sixth grade, he shrugged.

With a few days of resumption of antipsychotic medication, Mr. I. reported that his hallucinations were gone and that he felt less sad. Then he revealed that when he was in sixth grade his stepfather beat him and broke his arm. For as long as he could remember, his stepfather beat him constantly. He beat him badly at least twice weekly, and several times so badly that he had to be taken to hospital for injuries. His stepfather warned him to tell nobody.

In addition, he revealed that on the ward he was always sad and often cried and that he only slept about 4 hours per night, spending hours awake in bed thinking of his grandfather. He denied thoughts of suicide. Given this report, his psychiatrist prescribed paroxetine 20 mg daily with amitriptyline 50 mg at bedtime in addition to haloperidol.

Within a month of antidepressant treatment, Mr. I. was a diligent and cheerful patient-worker on the custodial crew. On the ward, he attended therapeutic groups more regularly, spruced himself up, and spontaneously greeted others with a smile. He was eager to leave the hospital and work full-time. Mr. I. was discharged with a diagnosis of major depressive disorder. He met some criteria for posttraumatic stress disorder (PTSD), but his psychiatrist failed to explore further to determine if he met full criteria.

4.6 AUDITORY HALLUCINATIONS AND TRAUMA

In the case presented in the previous section, Mr. I. initially reported episodic symptoms. These were two short episodes of time travel and confusion triggered by the stress of death of family members with, at least according to what he told fitness examiners, auditory hallucinations. His hallucinations at the time of his arrest could have been due to his use of cannabis (American Psychiatric Association, 2022a), as his psychiatrist initially believed. By "time travel" he seemed to be describing flashbacks (i.e., returning to the past). These episodes could best be explained as dissociative experiences. Flashbacks are characteristic of posttraumatic stress disorder (PTSD) and acute stress disorder (American Psychiatric Association, 2022b).

Later, Mr. I. revealed chronic, almost continuous hallucinations from childhood and a history of childhood physical abuse. A history of chronic hallucinations might bring to mind schizophrenia, but Mr. I. did not meet diagnostic criteria for that illness, if only because his sole symptom was hallucinations. His idea about time travel was not a delusion, not a fixed belief, because he described it as a foolish thing he imagined. In addition, onset of schizophrenia prior to adolescence is rare (American Psychiatric Association, 2022a).

If not schizophrenia, what diagnosis could account for his history? Could his hallucinations and history of abuse be related? Auditory hallucinations and other psychotic symptoms in children and adults are related to a history of childhood abuse. In a study of 2,232 twin children and their families (Arseneault et al., 2011), 12-year-old children who had experienced either bullying or physical abuse were 3.27 times as likely to report psychotic symptoms compared to those who experienced neither. Those who experienced both were 5.68 times more likely. Risks remained higher after controlling for other variables that could be related to psychosis in children. In a representative survey of 7,353 adults in England (Bebbington, 2011), self-reported childhood sexual abuse, particularly nonconsensual sexual intercourse, was strongly related to psychotic symptoms in adulthood.

Some adults who hallucinate have no diagnosable psychiatric illness; they are called "healthy voice hearers" because they experience persistent auditory hallucinations but do not need mental health care or suffer much distress. These individuals have a higher rate of lifetime trauma compared to healthy controls (Baumeister et al., 2017).

However, trauma exposure is associated with multiple psychiatric diagnoses in which psychotic symptoms can be manifest, such as substance abuse, depression with psychotic features, personality disorders, and especially trauma-related diagnoses such as PTSD (Compean and Hamner, 2019).

"Psychotic-like symptoms" such as hallucinations during times of stress have been described in people with borderline personality disorder (BPD) (American Psychiatric Association, 2022c).

But, according to one review (Cavelti et al., 2021), auditory hallucinations in adults with BPD are widespread, occurring in 29–50%, and are often more than transient. Comparing symptoms in people with schizophrenia to symptoms in people with BPD, hallucinations with BPD are more likely to start earlier in life (i.e., in adolescence). In addition, BPD patients show less delusional thinking, negative symptoms, and conceptual disorganization. When chronic hallucinations occur in people with BPD, some authors have attributed them to comorbid conditions, such as mood disorders and PTSD (Barnow et al., 2010).

In a study of PTSD, childhood trauma, lifetime trauma, and psychotic disorder in 328 adults, lifetime trauma was not significantly related to current psychotic disorder, but a history of childhood abuse was. Compared to adults with no or low levels of exposure to child abuse, those with significant child abuse exposure were 3.5 times as likely to be diagnosed with a current psychotic disorder. A PTSD diagnosis seemed to mediate the relationship between trauma and psychosis (Powers et al., 2016).

PTSD has been associated with auditory hallucinations and with other psychotic symptoms (Compean & Hamner, 2019; David et al., 1999). In one study of this association, combat veterans with PTSD and co-occurring auditory hallucinations and other psychotic symptoms did not usually also have thought disorder or inappropriate affect. Psychotic symptoms were significantly associated with major depressive disorder (David et al., 1999). In a community sample (Sareen et al., 2005), people with a lifetime diagnosis of PTSD were significantly more likely to endorse lifetime positive psychotic symptoms, particularly auditory hallucinations, compared to people without lifetime PTSD. Individuals with PTSD and psychotic symptoms were more likely to have other psychiatric disorders (including major depressive disorder and substance abuse) compared to individuals with PTSD and no psychotic symptoms, but the relationship between PTSD and psychosis remained after controlling for other psychiatric disorders.

REFERENCES

American Psychiatric Association. (2022a). Schizophrenia spectrum and other psychotic disorders. In *Diagnostic and Statistical Manual of Mental Disorders*, 5th ed., text revision, pp. 101–136. Washington, DC: American Psychiatric Association.

American Psychiatric Association. (2022b). Trauma- and stressor-related disorders. In *Diagnostic and Statistical Manual of Mental Disorders*, 5th ed., text revision, pp. 295–348. Washington, DC: American Psychiatric Association.

American Psychiatric Association. (2022c). Personality disorders. In *Diagnostic and Statistical Manual of Mental Disorders*, 5th ed., text revision, pp. 733–778. Washington, DC: American Psychiatric Association.

Arseneault, L., Cannon, M., Polanczyk, G., Moffit, T. E., & Caspi, A. (2011). Childhood trauma and children's emerging psychotic symptoms: A genetically sensitive longitudinal cohort study. *American Journal of Psychiatry* 168(1):65–72.

Barnow, S., Arens, E. A., Sieswerda, S., Dinu-Biringer, R., Spitzer, C., & Lang, S. (2010). Borderline personality disorder and psychosis: A review. *Current Psychiatry Reports* 12:186–195.

Baumeister, D., Sedgwick, O., Howes, O., & Peters, E. (2017). Auditory verbal hallucinations and continuum models of psychosis: A systematic review of the healthy voice-hearer literature. *Clinical Psychology Review* 51:125–141.

Bebbington, P., Jonas, S., Kuipers, E., King, M., Cooper, C., Brugha, T., . . . & Jenkins, R. (2011). Childhood sexual abuse and psychosis: Data from a cross-sectional national psychiatric survey in England. *British Journal of Psychiatry* 199:29–37.

Cavelti, M., Thompson, K., Chanen, A. M., & Kaess, M. (2021). Psychotic symptoms in borderline personality disorder: Developmental aspects. *Current Opinion in Psychology* 37:26–31.

Compean, E., & Hamner, M. (2019). Posttraumatic stress disorder with secondary psychotic features (PTSD-SP): Diagnostic and treatment challenges. *Progress in Neuropsychopharacology and Biological Psychiatry* 88:265–275.

David, D., Kutcher, G. S., Jackson, E., & Mellman, T. A. (1999). Psychotic symptoms in combat-related posttraumatic stress disorder. *Journal of Clinical Psychiatry* 60:29–32.

Powers, A., Fani, N., Cross, D., Ressler, K. J., & Bradley, B. (2016). Childhood trauma, PTSD and psychosis: Findings from a highly traumatized, minority sample. *Child Abuse and Neglect* 58: 111–118.

Sareen, J., Cox, B. J., Goodwin, R. D., & Asmundson, G. J. G. (2005). Co-occurrence of posttraumatic stress disorder with positive psychotic symptoms in a nationally representative sample. *Journal of Traumatic Stress* 18(4):313–322.

5

USING CLOZAPINE

This chapter reports on data demonstrating the superior efficacy of clozapine for multiple indications: with treatment-resistant schizophrenia and with violent behavior and suicidality in people with schizophrenia. It can also normalize hyponatremia due to psychogenic polydipsia and alleviate severe affective and borderline personality disorders. Cases illustrate improvement in two patients with schizophrenia and in one with major depressive disorder with psychotic features. The chapter also outlines potential adverse effects. Possible risks should be weighed against possible benefits while keeping in mind that psychiatric patients have a right to treatment that gives each a realistic chance of at least some improvement in their condition.

5.1 CASE J: A MAN WITH A PARTIAL RESPONSE

5.1.1 Case

Mr. J. was a man in his early 20s with long-standing behavior problems and paranoid delusions whose most recent admission to a state hospital was precipitated by an assault on a close relative. On the day he hit multiple staff members and patients, he was transferred to a smaller, specialized unit.

Interview

His treatment team met with Mr. J. soon after he arrived on the unit and then weekly to discuss his treatment plan and any questions or concerns he had. A few weeks after he arrived, his team leader asked him why he should take medication. He first said "Because you said so," but, with prodding, said because he heard voices and saw things. Mr. J. could not say what he had learned in his groups. What he did want to talk about, repeatedly and with urgency, was obtaining a bag of his favorite salty, spicy chips. Besides chips, his only request was to go home soon so he could see his family more often. He squirmed but managed to stay seated for 5–10 minutes, then gathered up momentum and bolted out of his chair.

History

Mr. J.'s first state psychiatric hospitalization occurred in his early teens when he was in a regular school with an individualized plan to address his learning disabilities. His mother noticed he had changed in the previous few months in that he had become irritable and claimed she wanted to hurt him. When he pushed and shoved her, he was admitted to a hospital. There he started fights with other children and voiced clear psychotic symptoms such as the belief that his food was poisoned and that people on TV were speaking directly to him. With antipsychotic medication, he was discharged home and to his school.

Mr. J. was hospitalized on many more occasions, though he was offered an array of outpatient services of increasing intensity. A second hospitalization occurred a few months after his first. On discharge, he started an intensive day program for adolescents, which helped him stay out of hospitals for more than a year. When it was clear he could not participate in his program, he moved to a residential treatment facility, where he stayed for several months but then returned to a state hospital. Despite an assisted outpatient treatment (AOT) order and an assertive community treatment (ACT) team, his psychiatric hospitalizations became more frequent and longer.

The latest of these hospitalizations occurred after he slapped his mother. His inpatient psychiatrist tried long-acting intramuscular medications and oral medications of different classes, with little success. Eventually he and Mr. J.'s mother convinced the young man to take clozapine. He showed some benefit but was inconsistently adherent, and, when he refused more doses than he accepted, he became more dangerous. His doctor tried to understand why he hit people, but Mr. J. could not explain or even use complete sentences.

Course of treatment

The small, specialized unit made fewer demands and provided Mr. J. more supervision and one-to-one attention. Though he was encouraged to attend groups and other programs, much of the day he spent pacing, and, as he paced, he sang or laughed out loud to himself. Given a chance, he masturbated openly and urinated on the floor. Ward staff found puddles of urine under his bed, in the corners of his room, and along the hallway leading to the bathroom. On some occasions, he stared at and talked to his reflection in a blank TV screen. Once he explained he was just looking at how cute he was. But another day he revealed that he heard the voice of a popular and sexy female movie star, so it was more likely he was hallucinating.

On this unit, with intense supervision, Mr. J. took every dose of clozapine his nurse offered. Though he still hallucinated, he did not hit anyone, rarely urinated on the floor, and attended some groups. He could not be discharged, but he was well enough to be transferred to a regular ward.

5.2 CLOZAPINE TREATMENT OF SCHIZOPHRENIA

5.2.1 Early history of clozapine use

Clozapine was a new and intriguing antipsychotic drug in the 1960s and early 1970s (Hippius, 1999), with distinctive pharmacologic properties (Kane et al., 1988). Its prospects took a dramatic turn in 1975, when 16 Finnish patients who were taking it developed granulocytopenia; 13 of these developed agranulocytosis and 8 died due to resulting infection (Kane et al., 1988). The drug was withdrawn from the market in countries where it was in clinical use and from clinical research in the United States (Kane et al., 1988). But after patients who had responded to clozapine relapsed (Hippius, 1999), the drug returned to limited, humanitarian use with intensive hematologic monitoring in the United States and other countries. Research interest in clozapine continued as studies published between 1974 and 1988 suggested that clozapine was more efficacious than other agents (Kane et al., 1988).

5.2.2 Trial in treatment-resistant patients

A turning point for clozapine was the 1988 publication of a double-blind comparison with chlorpromazine in 319 treatment-resistant patients (Kane et al., 1988). This trial was based on the premise that the apparent greater risk of clozapine could be justified in carefully monitored patients who had not responded adequately to other antipsychotics.

Treatment resistance was defined by history of response, current condition, and response determined prospectively. Historical criteria were at least three trials in the previous 5 years with agents from at least two antipsychotic drug classes at substantial doses (equivalent to at least 1,000 mg/day chlorpromazine) without significant symptom improvement and no period of good functioning within those 5 years.

Patients who met the historical criteria were also required to demonstrate at least moderate severity of current symptoms as measured by Brief Psychiatric Rating Scale (BPRS) (Overall & Gorham, 1962) total and psychotic symptom scores and Clinical Global Impression (CGI), a clinical measure of overall severity of symptoms (Guy, 1976).

To demonstrate treatment resistance prospectively, study participants who met the above criteria entered a 6-week trial of haloperidol with benztropine. To be considered a haloperidol responder, patients had to show at least a 20% decrease in total BPRS score and a CGI rating of mildly ill, or a total BPRS score of 35 or less. Patients who responded to haloperidol were not continued in the study.

Patients who continued the study were treated with either chlorpromazine and benztropine or clozapine at substantial doses over 6 weeks. Patients were monitored with regular lab testing and evaluations of psychopathology with BPRS and a nurses' scale measuring ward behavior. Criteria for response in this trial were the same as those in the haloperidol trial, that is, at least a 20% decrease in total BPRS score and a CGI rating of mildly ill, or a total BPRS score of 35 or less

From the first week of treatment, greater improvement with clozapine was obvious. Of the patients who completed at least 1 week of the drug comparison, 4% of patients on chlorpromazine met criteria for improvement, while 30% of clozapine patients did so. Improvement in BPRS total score and CGI was about three times greater in clozapine patients. Clozapine performed significantly better than chlorpromazine in the treatment of positive and negative symptoms and in ratings of ward behavior. No patient developed agranulocytosis.

Even with clozapine many patients did not respond well. Seventy percent of patients on clozapine did not meet criteria for improvement. A recent estimate is that at least 40% of patients treated with clozapine will have a suboptimal response (Meyer & Stahl, 2020a).

5.2.3 FDA approval

In 1989, on the strength of the Kane and colleagues study, the US Food and Drug Administration (FDA) approved the use of clozapine for treatment refractory patients with schizophrenia and for those who could not tolerate other antipsychotics. The drug was approved with a requirement for routine white blood cell and/or absolute neutrophil count monitoring (Meyer & Stahl, 2020b). This requirement was eliminated February 24, 2025, although the FDA still recommends that prescribers monitor patients' absolute neutrophil counts (US Food and Drug Administration, 2025).

5.2.4 Use with patients with schizophrenia

The American Psychiatric Association (APA) Practice Guideline for the Treatment of Patients with Schizophrenia (American Psychiatric Association, 2021) recommends clozapine for patients who are treatment-resistant but does not define resistance. A definition of treatment resistance (Howe et al., 2017) is similar to the criteria in the 1988 Kane study in that it requires past treatment of a similar duration and with similar dosages and number of antipsychotics. Like the Kane study criteria, the definition requires at least moderate current functional impairment and symptom severity measured by a standardized rating scale. In contrast, instead of a prospective trial, the definition requires methods to establish adherence; one is obtaining antipsychotic plasma levels at least once. Some patients whom clinicians identify as treatment-resistant are not responding because they are not consistently taking medication as prescribed.

Since the time of the Kane study, there has been a movement to broaden eligibility for clozapine. Instead of three trials of antipsychotics at 1,000 mg/day chlorpromazine equivalents, two trials at moderate doses (equivalent to 300–1,000 mg/day chlorpromazine) are considered sufficient. In addition, treatment-resistance can be viewed as a continuous, not categorical concept. Most patients seen as unresponsive are suboptimal responders of varying degrees (Nakagome & Mogami, 2012).

5.2.5 Underuse in United States

Use of clozapine is widely variable between countries. For example, a 2006 survey found it was used in 32% of all patients taking antipsychotics in China. Chinese guidelines highly recommend but do not require routine blood testing (Wang & Li, 2012). In that country, clozapine is cheap and often used as a first-line agent (Si et al., 2012).

Clozapine is prescribed much less in the United States, at rates well below rates of treatment resistance, which are estimated to be 20–30%. Between 2006 and 2009, in all state Medicaid programs, clozapine accounted for 4.8% of total antipsychotics started in patients with schizophrenia. However, states have varied widely in clozapine initiation, with the highest rate in South Dakota at 15.6%, and the lowest in Louisiana at 2.0% (Olfson et al., 2016).

Psychiatrists and other practitioners may be underutilizing clozapine because they are not familiar with its use and cannot turn to colleagues with more experience; because they have concerns about the drug's safety (Cohen, 2014); or because they do not appreciate its superior efficacy. In the past, another reason could have been inflexible requirements for hematologic monitoring.

Clozapine use can change. One state hospital system made coordinated efforts to increase clozapine use. With educational supports, a telephone help line, testimonials from patients, and tracking of progress, state hospital practitioners started more patients on clozapine. The increase in the rate of new starts was more than three times the increase in non-state settings (Carruthers et al., 2016).

State hospitals often treat patients likely to benefit from clozapine and can be ideal settings for treatment initiation. They can offer close patient monitoring, medical backup, collegial consultation, and continuing education. Studies of clozapine-treated state hospital patients have found life-changing improvement. In Oregon (Wilson & Claussen, 1995), a review of records of the first 100 state hospital patients to receive clozapine—individuals who were chronically ill and poor responders to other treatments—discovered that, after 18 months, 45 were much improved and 18 were somewhat improved. Forty patients had been discharged. In Texas (Reid, 1999), a group of state hospital patients with schizophrenia who were taking clozapine were compared to a matched group taking other antipsychotic drugs. Over the course of 4 years, patients on clozapine required appreciably fewer days in hospital than those on other antipsychotic drugs.

5.2.6 Schizophrenia and aggression

Researchers in Oregon (Wilson & Clausen, 1995) also noticed a decrease in violent episodes in the first 6 months of clozapine use. Investigators in Connecticut found that state hospital patients treated with clozapine compared to patients treated with other antipsychotics were significantly less disruptive (Essock et al., 2000). These studies were open and not designed to explore clozapine's effect on violent inpatients.

A study so designed was a 12-week randomized, double-blind comparison of clozapine, olanzapine, and haloperidol in the treatment of aggression and psychiatric symptoms in 110 violent state hospital patients with schizophrenia or schizoaffective disorder in New York (Krakowski et al., 2006). The study took place on a research unit where nursing staff frequently monitored each patient for physical and verbal aggression and aggression against property. Change in aggression scores over time was statistically significant between treatment groups. Total aggression and physical aggression scores were significantly lower for treatment with clozapine than for treatment with olanzapine or haloperidol. Scores were lower for treatment with olanzapine than with haloperidol. This study is evidence for a specific anti-aggressive effect of clozapine. It did not find a superior antipsychotic effect, but that was not its purpose; its subjects were not treatment-resistant.

The APA Practice Guideline (American Psychiatric Association, 2021) suggests clozapine for patients with schizophrenia who are at risk for violence when other treatments have not been successful.

5.2.7 Schizophrenia and suicidality

A 2005 review (Palmer et al., 2005) estimated the lifetime rate for completed suicide among people with schizophrenia at 4.9%. Estimated lifetime rates of suicide attempts are much higher, 25–50% (Meltzer, 2001).

Use of clozapine was associated with a fivefold decrease in the rate of completed suicide among people with schizophrenia in the Texas public mental health system (Reid, 1999).

Use of clozapine is also associated with decreased rates of suicidality (i.e., suicidal thoughts and attempts). The International Suicide Prevention Trial (Meltzer et al., 2003) was a prospective trial comparing the effects of clozapine and olanzapine on suicidality. Of 958 subjects with schizophrenia or schizoaffective illness, 477 were treated with olanzapine and 479 with clozapine. All were at high risk for suicidality due to either current suicidal ideas, recent command hallucinations to self-harm, or a history of suicide attempts or of hospitalizations to prevent attempts. Patients were followed over the course of 2 years with regular monitoring of suicidal thinking and behavior. Compared to patients treated with olanzapine, patients treated with clozapine had significantly fewer suicide attempts (34 vs. 55) and significantly fewer hospitalizations to prevent suicide (82 vs. 107). The rate per year of suicide attempts was 5.6% for clozapine patients and 8.5% for olanzapine patients.

The APA Practice Guideline (American Psychiatric Association, 2021) recommends clozapine for patients at risk for suicide when other treatments have not been successful.

5.2.8 Polydipsia and hyponatremia

Polyuria and polydipsia have been described in state hospital patients with schizophrenia at least since 1935 (Sleeper, 1935). Many years later, two surveys of state hospital patients resulted in estimates that at least 20% had polydipsia and resulting polyuria (Verghese et al., 1996).

Polydipsia has been defined as drinking 3 liters or more of fluid per day. After drug and medical causes have been ruled out, the etiology is unknown, but the condition is associated with schizophrenia, although not exclusively (Verghese et al., 1996). In one review of clinical studies and case reports (Kirino et al., 2020), 70% of patients with polydipsia were diagnosed with schizophrenia and 26% with mental retardation.

Though the condition is less common than polydipsia, a significant proportion of polydipsic patients cannot excrete excess water and so develop hyponatremia (Vieweg & Leadbetter, 1997). Hyponatremia can be chronic. It may produce no obvious symptoms (Verghese et al., 1996). Or, it may produce confusion, ataxia, slurred speech (Koczapski & Millson, 1989), delirium, seizures, and coma (Vieweg & Leadbetter, 1997). In an observational study of eight patients (Koczapski & Millson, 1989), the severity of symptoms was related to the amount and speed of change in sodium levels rather than the absolute levels. Death can result, as described in five patients from Western State Hospital in Virginia (Vieweg et al., 1985).

Fluid restriction has been the standard treatment, but it requires confinement to a hospital with close monitoring of fluid intake and does not seem to influence the excessive urge to drink water (Verghese et al., 1996). Fluid intake can be measured by daily weight gain. In a study of eight hospitalized patients with polydipsia, serum sodium was strongly correlated with percentage increase in weight from morning to evening. During the night patients always excreted water and lost weight (Delva & Crammer, 1988).

Clozapine can affect polydipsia and allow hospital discharge. Eight patients with hyponatremia and treatment-resistant schizophrenia at a state hospital in Illinois were treated openly with clozapine over 18 weeks (Canuso & Goldman, 1999). With clozapine 300 mg/day both urine and plasma osmolality, measures of water balance that are related to serum sodium level, significantly increased and plasma osmolality normalized. Doses of 600 mg and 900 mg were not associated with further significant increases. All eight patients were discharged from the hospital on clozapine within 3 months of completing the study, after an average of 5 years continuous stay.

Because the severity of symptoms is related to the degree and speed of change in sodium levels (Koczapski & Millson, 1989) clinicians should be vigilant when discontinuing clozapine in patients with a history of polydipsia. Abrupt discontinuation can lead to a rapid change in sodium levels that could be lethal. Similarly, rapid correction of hyponatremia with hypertonic saline can produce a potentially fatal neurologic condition, central pontine myelinolysis or osmotic dysmyelination (Pearce, 2009).

REFERENCES

American Psychiatric Association. (2021). Pharmacotherapy In *Practice Guideline for the Treatment of Patients with Schizophrenia*, 3rd ed. Eds. G. A. Keepers et al., pp. 33–118. Washington, DC: American Psychiatric Association.

Canuso, C. M., & Goldman, M. B. (1999). Clozapine restores water balance in schizophrenic patients with polydipsia-hyponatremia syndrome. *Journal of Neuropsychiatry and Clinical Neuroscience* 11(1):86–90.

Carruthers, J., Radigan, M., Erlich, M. D., Gu, G., Wang, R., Frimfong, E. Y. . . . & Stroup, T. S. (2016). An initiative to improve clozapine prescribing in New York State. *Psychiatric Services* 67(4):369–371.

Cohen, D. (2014). Prescribers fear as a major side-effect of clozapine. *Acta Psychiatrica Scandinavica* 130:154–155.

Delva, N. J., & Crammer, J. L. (1988). Polydipsia in chronic psychiatric patients: Body weight and serum sodium. *British Journal of Psychiatry* 152:242–245.

Essock, S. M., Frisman, L. K., Covell, N. H., & Hargreaves, W. (2000). Cost-effectiveness of clozapine compared with conventional antipsychotic medications for patients in state hospitals. *Archives of General Psychiatry* 57:987–994.

Guy, W. (1976). Clinical global impressions. In *ECDEU Assessment Manual for Psychopharmacology*, revised, pp. 216–222. Rockville, MD: National Institute of Mental Health.

Hippius, H. (1999). A historical perspective of clozapine. *Journal of Clinical Psychiatry* 60(suppl 12):22–23.

Howes, O. D., McCutcheon, R., Agid, O., de Bartolomeis, A., van Beveren, N. J. M., Birnbaum, M. L., . . . & Correll, C. U. (2017). Treatment-resistant schizophrenia: Treatment Response and Resistance in Psychosis (TRRIP) Working Group consensus guidelines on diagnosis and terminology. *American Journal of Psychiatry* 174(3):216–229.

Kane, J. M., Honigfeld, G., Singer, J., & Meltzer H. (1988). Clozapine for the treatment-resistant schizophrenia: A double-blind comparison with chlorpromazine. *Archives of General Psychiatry* 45:789–796.

Kirino, S., Sakuma, M., Misawa, F., Fujii, Y., Uchida, H., Mimura, M., & Takeuchi, H. (2020). Relationship between polydipsia and antipsychotics: A systematic review of clinical studies and case reports. *Progress in Neuropsychopharmacology and Biological Psychiatry* 96:109756. doi: 10.1016/j.pnpbp.2019.109756. Epub 2019 Aug 28.

Koczapski, A. B., & Millson, R. C. (1989). Individual differences in serum sodium levels in schizophrenia men with self-induced water intoxication. *American Journal of Psychiatry* 146(12):1614–1615.

Krakowski, M. I., Czovor, P., Citrome, L., Bark, N., & Cooper, T. B. (2006). Atypical antipsychotic agents in the treatment of violent patients with schizophrenia and schizoaffective disorder. *Archives of General Psychiatry* 63:622–629.

Meltzer, H. Y. (2001). Treatment of suicidality in schizophrenia. *Annals of the New York Academy of Science* 932:44–58; discussion 58–60.

Meltzer, H. Y., Alphs, L., Green, A. I., Altamura, A. C., Anand, R., Bertoldi, A., . . . & Potkin, S. (2003). Clozapine treatment for suicidality in schizophrenia: International Suicide Prevention Trial (InterSePT). *Archives of General Psychiatry* 60:82–91.

Meyer, J. M., & Stahl, S. M. (2020a). Addressing clozapine positive symptom nonresponse in schizophrenia spectrum patients. In *The Clozapine Handbook*, pp. 44–89. Cambridge: Cambridge University Press.

Meyer, J. M., & Stahl, S. M. (2020b). Understanding hematologic monitoring and benign ethnic neutropenia. In *The Clozapine Handbook*, pp. 114–137. Cambridge: Cambridge University Press.

Nakagome, K., & Mogami, T. (2012). Treatment-resistant schizophrenia. In *Clinical Manual for Treatment of Schizophrenia*. Eds. J. Lauriello & S. Pallanti, pp. 358–359. Washington, DC: American Psychiatric Publishing.

Olfson, M., Gerhard, T., Crystal, S., & Stroup, S. (2016). Clozapine for schizophrenia: State variation in evidence-based practice. *Psychiatric Services* 67(2):152.

Overall, J. E., & Gorham, D. R. (1962). The Brief Psychiatric Rating Scale. *Psychological Reports* 10(3):799–812.

Palmer, B. A., Pankratz, V. S., & Bostwick, J. M. (2005). The lifetime risk of suicide in schizophrenia: A reexamination. *Archives of General Psychiatry* 62(3):247–253.

Pearce, J. M. S. (2009). Central pontine myelinolysis. *European Neurology* 61:59–62.

Reid, W. H. (1999). New vs. old antipsychotics: The Texas experience. *Journal of Clinical Psychiatry* 60(suppl 1):23–24.

Si, T.-M., Zhang, Y.-s., Shu, L., Li, K.-Q., Liu, X.-H., Mei, Q.-Y., . . . & Yu, X. (2012). Use of Clozapine for the Treatment of Schizophrenia: Findings of the 2006 Research on the China Psychotropic Prescription Studies. *Clinical Psychopharmacology and Neuroscience* 10(2):99–104.

Sleeper, F. H. (1935). Investigation of polyuria in schizophrenia. *American Journal of Psychiatry* 91:1019–1031.

US Food and Drug Administration. (2025). Frequently asked questions | Clozapine REMS modification. Accessed from: https://www.fda.gov/drugs/postmarket-drug-safety-information-patients-and-providers/frequently-asked-questions-clozapine-rems-modification.

Verghese, C., de Leon, J., & Josiassen, R. C. (1996). Problems and progress in the diagnosis and treatment of polydipsia and hyponatremia. *Schizophrenia Bulletin* 22(3):455–464.

Vieweg, W. V., & Leadbetter, R. A. (1997). Polydipsia-hyponatraemia syndrome: Epidemiology, clinical features and treatment. *Drug Therapy* 7(2):121–138.

Vieweg, W. V. R., David, J. J., Rowe, W. T., Wampler, G. J., Burns, W. J., & Spradlin, W. W. (1985). Death from self-induced water intoxication among patients with schizophrenic disorders. *Journal of Nervous and Mental Disease* 173(3):161–165.

Wang, C., & Li, L. (2012). Proper use of clozapine: Experiences in China. *Shanghai Archives of Psychiatry* 24(2):108–109.

Wilson, W. H., & Claussen, A. M. (1995). 18-month outcome of clozapine treatment for 100 patients in a state psychiatric hospital. *Psychiatric Services* 46(4):386–389.

5.3 CASE K: A MAN WITH A LOW NEUTROPHIL COUNT

5.3.1 Case

Mr. K. was an African American man in his early 20s who was transferred from a community hospital to a state psychiatric hospital.

History

This young man was first admitted for psychiatric treatment to a local community hospital in his late teens. A few months after his first discharge his parents brought him to the emergency room (ER) of the same hospital because their son would not leave their apartment and had stopped eating. In the ER, he revealed that he saw angels and demons in his room and heard the TV talking to him.

Mr. K.'s treatment at the community hospital did not ameliorate his condition. Just prior to his transfer to a state hospital doctors wrote that he was hallucinating and nearly mute with catatonic features, such as muscle rigidity, despite treatment with multiple antipsychotic agents at adequate doses.

Course of treatment

At the state hospital Mr. K. paced the hallways flapping one hand, undressed in public, and hit another patient. Later he became rigid, resisted efforts to move his limbs, and refused to eat or drink. He was transferred to a ward with a small population and started on clozapine. However, a few days later, his neutrophil count, which was low before clozapine was started, dropped lower. His dismayed psychiatrist discontinued clozapine and started another antipsychotic.

As a result, his treatment at the state hospital was stymied by fear of granulocytopenia. Mr. K. mostly sat at a distance from other patients, in the same chair, planted in front of a television, with an attendant seated a few feet away. He would intermittently clench his fists and stiffen his neck and occasionally made requests of staff members he knew. He ate enough, but barely.

On interview with a senior psychiatrist who came to review his treatment, Mr. K. turned away and met most questions with silence. When he did speak, he showed no feeling and said only "OK," that he was OK. With the advice and encouragement of colleagues, Mr. K.'s treating psychiatrist restarted clozapine.

While on a low dose of clozapine Mr. K. punched a hole in the wall, knocked over an attendant, and went after another patient with his fists. A brave nurse obtained blood so clozapine could be continued and increased. Within a few weeks of ongoing clozapine, Mr. K. quit attacking people.

After 8 weeks on clozapine he was gaining weight on his regular diet and asking for snacks. The ward clinicians and attendants had gained confidence that he would not attack someone, so his psychiatrist stopped assigning an attendant to sit with him, watching constantly. Still, he spent much time by himself, in the same seat, and did not initiate conversation except to ask for the television remote control. When approached, he spoke in logical short sentences.

By 12 weeks on clozapine, Mr. K. was transferred to a ward with a larger population. Soon he joined a few therapeutic groups and ventured outdoors to shoot some baskets. Throughout this, his second trial of clozapine, his neutrophil count did not drop.

5.3.2 Comment

Because psychiatrists treating Mr. K. were overly cautious, they were underutilizing clozapine. At the time, physicians were aware that baseline low neutrophil counts can be normal among some groups of people, but blood monitoring requirements did not take into account this phenomena. The US Food and Drug Administration (FDA) requirements for monitoring the use of clozapine have changed multiple times over the past several years. In 2015, the FDA issued new guidelines for patients with benign ethnic neutropenia, a normal variant in some ethnic groups, particularly people of African descent (Meyer & Stahl, 2020). With a new perspective and collegial support, Mr. K.'s treatment could move forward. While he did not have a complete remission of his illness, his functioning improved greatly.

REFERENCE

Meyer, J. M., & Stahl, S. M. (2020). Understanding hematologic monitoring and benign ethnic neutropenia. In *The Clozapine Handbook* pp. 114–139. Cambridge: Cambridge University Press.

5.4 ADVERSE EFFECTS

Clozapine has exceptional potential to benefit certain groups of patients, but it also carries the risk of some atypical adverse effects and complications. Some affect patients' quality of life and can contribute to nonadherence, while a few can be dangerous. What follows is a general overview of clozapine's possible adverse effects. It is not exhaustive and is not meant to substitute for careful reading of a psychopharmacology textbook and collegial consultation.

5.4.1 Compared to other antipsychotics

Clozapine is not likely to cause some of the adverse effects common to other antipsychotics. It is not likely to cause extrapyramidal symptoms (EPS) or elevated prolactin levels (American Psychiatric Association, 2021). Tardive dyskinesia is rare with clozapine use (Meyer & Stahl, 2020a).

The drug is, however, associated with different adverse effects common to other antipsychotics, with some variations in frequency and severity. Both clozapine and olanzapine are highly likely to cause metabolic abnormalities and QT prolongation. Compared to olanzapine, clozapine is more often associated with seizures and orthostasis. It is similar to chlorpromazine and other low-potency first-generation drugs in that it often causes sedation and anticholinergic effects, and it is similar to chlorpromazine in that it can cause tachycardia (American Psychiatric Association, 2021).

Clinicians should be alert to hematologic adverse effects, but, according to a summary of available evidence, the risk of neutropenia and of severe neutropenia is not greater with clozapine than it is with other antipsychotics (Myles et al., 2019). Another review (Myles et al., 2018) concluded that the incidence of clozapine-associated severe neutropenia was 0.9% and the incidence of death related to this condition was 0.013%. The incidence of severe neutropenia peaked at 1 month of treatment and fell to negligible levels after 1 year.

The US Food and Drug Administration (FDA) no longer expects psychiatrists and nurse practitioners to participate in the risk evaluation and mitigation strategies (REMS) program for clozapine or to report results of absolute neutrophil count (ANC) blood tests before pharmacies dispense clozapine. The FDA still recommends that prescribers monitor patients' ANC according to the monitoring frequencies described in the drug's prescribing information (US Food and Drug Administration, 2025a).

An international panel of clozapine prescribers and expert academics (Siskind et al., 2026) reached a consensus recommending ANC monitoring weekly for the first 18 weeks of clozapine treatment, then every 4 weeks until 2 years after initiation of clozapine. After 2 years, hematologic testing should be completed annually.

5.4.2 Particularly concerning side effects

Gastrointestinal hypomotility, often manifested by constipation, is much more common and potentially more dangerous than severe neutropenia. Clozapine affects transit time through the colon far more than other antipsychotic agents that are known to produce constipation. The worst complication of gastrointestinal hypomotility, paralytic ileus, has a mortality rate of 15–27.5%, considerably higher than the rate for severe neutropenia (Meyer & Stahl, 2020b).

Sialorrhea can be seen with other antipsychotics (American Psychiatric Association, 2021) but is very common with clozapine. In the Kane and colleagues (1988) study comparing clozapine to chlorpromazine, sialorrhea occurred in 13% of 126 clozapine patients and 1% of 142 chlorpromazine patients. It occurred in 31% of 842 patients across multiple studies (US Food and Drug Administration, 2025b, pp. 16–17). Sialorrhea and sedation can increase the risk of aspiration pneumonia. Infection and cessation of cigarette smoking will increase blood levels of clozapine and cause more sedation (Correll et al., 2022). Pneumonia is one of the most important causes of mortality with clozapine, much more so than agranulocytosis (De Leon et al., 2020).

Fever may occur in about 20% of patients in the first 8 weeks of clozapine treatment and is often benign. Benign fever is not a reason to permanently stop clozapine, though it may be held pending the results of a fever workup (Meyers & Stahl, 2020c). One possible cause of fever is clozapine-related myocarditis. Myocarditis can present with nonspecific flu-like symptoms such as malaise, myalgia, pleuritic chest pain, and low-grade fevers (US Food and Drug Administration, 2025b, p. 29). The incidence of myocarditis is controversial, with a range of 0.1% to 3%, with higher rates found in Australia. It is fatal if not recognized and clozapine stopped (Meyers & Stahl, 2020c).

5.4.3 Prescribing clozapine

Before prescribing, any drugs that share clozapine's adverse effects should be discontinued or their doses minimized. Clozapine is highly anticholinergic, so other anticholinergic drugs can be risky. Clozapine can be sedating, so benzodiazepines and other sedating drugs should be tapered off as much as possible.

Clozapine adverse effects and therapeutic effects are related to plasma levels. With twice-daily or bedtime-only dosing, blood should be drawn in the morning after a bedtime dose and before any morning dose. This is a 12-hour trough level (Meyer & Stahl, 2020d). The minimum therapeutic level is 350 ng/mL, while levels greater than 600 ng/mL are associated with greater risk of some adverse effects (e.g., seizures). Factors that elevate clozapine levels are female gender, older age, Asian and South Asian descent, inflammation, obesity, and rapid titration (Correll et al., 2022).

Clozapine drug levels are also affected by drug–drug interactions. Certain drugs will inhibit or induce the particular cytochrome P450 isozymes by which clozapine is metabolized. Inhibitors will increase clozapine levels while inducers will decrease them. Strong inhibitors are fluvoxamine and ciprofloxacin. If clozapine is used with these drugs, its dose should be decreased to one-third the original dose. Strong inducers are carbamazepine, phenytoin, St. John's wort, and rifampin. Concomitant use of clozapine and these drugs is not recommended (US Food and Drug Administration, 2025b, p. 1).

Titration schedules should be individualized based on tolerability and the urgency of need for treatment (e.g., with violent patients) and not according to a fixed, standard schedule. A low starting dose can be calming and demonstrate to the patient some benefit. Starting at a dose that the patient cannot tolerate may lead to patient refusal. A medication that a patient cannot tolerate and refuses to continue has failed.

To boost chances of adherence, address adverse effects such as constipation and sialorrhea early (Meyer & Stahl, 2020d). Frequent follow-up, especially close to the time of clozapine initiation, is recommended. Expert consensus guidelines (Siskind et al., 2026) call for monitoring for adverse drug reactions at the time ANC testing is completed for the first 2 years of clozapine treatment, then every 3 months afterward. The guidelines present a thorough list of possible adverse effects for regular checks: metabolic syndrome, constipation and intestinal hypomotility, gastroesophageal reflux, sialorrhea, drooling and choking, sedation, nocturnal enuresis and urinary incontinence, dizziness and orthostatic hypotension, tachycardia, sleep apnea, seizures and myoclonus, obsessive-compulsive disorder symptoms, sexual dysfunction, and signs and symptoms suggestive of pneumonia or heart failure.

Before judging its success a clozapine trial should continue for at least 3 months after attainment of therapeutic plasma levels (Howes et al., 2017). If possible, discontinuation should be slow because abrupt discontinuation can cause cholinergic rebound, with profuse sweating, headache, nausea, vomiting, and diarrhea (US Food and Drug Administration, 2025b, p. 14).

REFERENCES

American Psychiatric Association. (2021). Pharmacotherapy. In *Practice Guideline for the Treatment of Patients with Schizophrenia*, 3rd ed. pp. 33–118. Washington, DC: American Psychiatric Publishing.

Correll, C. U., Agid, O., Crespo-Facorro, B., de Bartolomeis, A., Fagiolini, A., Seppala, N., & Howe, O. D. (2022). A guideline and checklist for initiating and managing clozapine treatment in patients with treatment-resistant schizophrenia. *CNS Drugs* 36:659–679.

de Leon, J., Ruan, C.-J., Schoretsanitios, G., & De las Cuevas, C. (2020). A rational use of clozapine based on adverse drug reactions, pharmacokinetics, and clinical pharmacopsychology. *Psychotherapy and Psychosomatics* 8.9(4):200–214.

Howes, O. D., McCutcheon, R., Agid, O., de Bartolomeis, A., van Beveren, N. J. M., Birnbaum M. L., . . . & Correll C. U. (2017). Treatment-resistant schizophrenia: Treatment Response and Resistance in Psychosis (TRRIP) Working Group consensus guidelines on diagnosis and terminology. *American Journal of Psychiatry* 174(3):216–229.

Kane, J. M., Honigfeld, G., Singer, J., & Meltzer, H. (1988). Clozapine for the treatment-resistant schizophrenia: A double-blind comparison with chlorpromazine. *Archives of General Psychiatry* 45:789–796.

Meyer, J. M., & Stahl, S. M. (2020a). Managing enuresis and incontinence, priapism, venous thromboembolism, neuroleptic malignant syndrome, tardive dyskinesia and obsessive compulsive disorder. In *The Clozapine Handbook*, pp. 242–257. Cambridge: Cambridge University Press.

Meyer, J. M., & Stahl, S. M. (2020b). Managing constipation. In *The Clozapine Handbook*, pp. 140–156. Cambridge: Cambridge University Press.

Meyer, J. M., & Stahl, S. M. (2020c). Fever, myocarditis, interstitial nephritis, DRESS, serositis, and cardiomyopathy. In *The Clozapine Handbook*, pp. 224–241. Cambridge: Cambridge University Press.

Meyer, J. M., & Stahl, S. M. (2020d). Initiating clozapine. In *The Clozapine Handbook*, pp. 60–77. Cambridge: Cambridge University Press.

Myles, N., Myles, H., Xia, S., Large, M., Bird, R., Galletly, C., . . . & Siskind, D. (2019). A meta-analysis of controlled studies comparing the association between clozapine and other antipsychotic medications and the development of neutropenia. *Australia and New Zealand Journal of Psychiatry* 5.3(5):403–412.

Myles, N., Myles, H., Xia, S., Large, M., Kisely, S., Galletly, C., . . . & Siskind, D. (2018). Meta-analysis examining the epidemiology of clozapine-associated neutropenia. *Acta Psychiatrica Scandanavica* 13.8(2):101–109.

Siskind, D., Northwood, K., Pillinger, T., Chan, S., Correll, C., Cotes, R., . . . & McCutcheon, R. (2026). Absolute neutrophil count and adverse drug reaction monitoring during clozapine treatment: Consensus guidelines rom a global Delphi panel. *Lancet Psychiatry* 13:77–86.

US Food and Drug Administration. (2025a). Frequently asked questions | Clozapine REMS modification. Accessed on November 15, 2025, from: https://www.fda.gov/drugs/postmarket-drug-safety-information-patients-and-providers/frequently-asked-questions-clozapine-rems-modification

US Food and Drug Administration. (2025b). Clozaril full prescribing information, revised 6/2025. Accessed on November 15, 2025, https://www.accessdata.fda.gov/drugsatfda_docs/label/2025/019758s107lbl.pdf#

5.5 CASE L: A SEVERELY DEPRESSED MAN RESPONDS TO CLOZAPINE

Case 5.1

Mr. L. was a man in his 60s who was transferred to a state hospital from a community hospital's psychiatric inpatient service.

Interview

When Mr. L. first arrived at the hospital, he said nothing. He sat stooped over in a chair, barely moving. He stared straight into his psychiatrist's eyes, but said nothing. He said nothing to internists who later examined him, nothing to any staff. For a minute during his psychiatric exam it seemed he was trying to say something, but he did not. He would not even shake his head in response to yes/no questions.

History

This man had been depressed for more than 30 years; he had multiple hospital admissions, usually separated by a year or more, and multiple overdose attempts. His hospital stays regularly ended with discharge to his apartment and the care of his outpatient psychiatrist. Two hospital stays characterize his illness and treatment.

Before one admission many years earlier, Mr. L. was living alone, with no social contacts except members of his support group and his dog. He was convinced that while his dog was well-liked, he was shunned and that members of his support group had turned against him. He feared his food was poisoned and so ate little. After inpatient treatment showed some success and discharge plans moved forward, he feared and resisted leaving the hospital.

A second admission occurred when, after the death of his dog, Mr. L. became more symptomatic. He was more guilt-ridden, more tearful, and intermittently suicidal. Once in the hospital he felt protected and wanted to stay, but he was seen as clinging and demanding, and, after about 2 months in hospital, he was discharged to his apartment.

Before his most recent community hospital stay, Mr. L. was found in his apartment unresponsive and surrounded by several empty pill bottles. Inpatient clinicians provided extended, vigorous treatment, first with ECT, which was ineffective, and then with antidepressant and antipsychotic agents, which were no more effective. Then they transferred him to a state hospital.

Course of treatment

At the state hospital Mr. L. needed intensive nursing care and supervision. Ward attendants dressed and spoon-fed him. Nurses monitored a catheter inserted into his bladder to alleviate urinary retention. When night attendants found him aimlessly wandering the ward, they returned him to his bed. While he communicated very little verbally, what Mr. L. expressed in writing was delusional.

Clozapine, with its highly anticholinergic properties, could have worsened his urinary retention. Therefore, he was first treated for his enlarged prostate, and then clozapine was added to the two antidepressants he was taking at the community hospital. Gradually, his face appeared more relaxed, he quit wandering at night, and he spoke more. He responded to his psychiatrist with one or two words, saying he felt better and did not think of suicide. Later he said that speaking with others made him very uncomfortable. With time, he spoke full sentences. He worried about money: about nonexistent debts, about how he would pay for his needs, even about how he would pay for the snacks he ate on the ward. While he still needed adult diapers, he used the toilet to evacuate his bowels. Four months after Mr. L. started clozapine, he could shower and dress himself with reminders and supervision and had made contact with his family.

Some weeks later, it seemed Mr. L.'s improvement had leveled off. He said he felt a little anxious, alone and angry, angry mostly at himself for not having made much of his life. Members of his treatment team encouraged him to attend off-ward therapeutic groups, but he did not. Neuropsychological testing, completed by a hospital psychologist, demonstrated poor memory and executive functioning, and, consequently, difficulty in planning and organization. These results supported a diagnosis of unspecified neurocognitive disorder in addition to major depressive disorder with psychotic features, recurrent. Because he believed he could not care for himself, Mr. L. agreed to discharge to a nursing home.

5.6 MOOD AND BORDERLINE PERSONALITY DISORDERS

Data to support the use of clozapine in the treatment of affective disorders and borderline personality disorder (BPD) is not of the same quality as data to support its use in patients with schizophrenia. Some available information comes from large studies of real-world practice using nationwide databases. These provide evidence that clozapine treatment of these disorders is associated with fewer psychiatric hospitalizations. Other information comes from small, open trials with severely ill hospitalized patients. These show hopeful but not conclusive results.

5.6.1 Major depressive disorder with psychosis

Using nationwide records of adults in Finland and Sweden diagnosed with major depressive disorder with psychotic features, investigators (Taipale et al., 2024) compared the likelihood of psychiatric hospitalization within the same person during periods of use versus non-use of particular medications. They found that, compared to both use of quetiapine and to no antipsychotic treatment, use of clozapine and of any long-acting injectable (LAI) was associated with decreased risk of hospitalization.

5.6.2 Bipolar disorder

In an observational study similar to that of treatment of major depressive disorder with psychotic features (Lahteenvuo et al., 2023), investigators searched Finnish nationwide databases for all adults diagnosed with bipolar disorder. The five medications associated with lowest risk of psychiatric admissions were three LAIs, lithium, and clozapine.

In Denmark, investigators used nationwide records to compare the number and length of psychiatric hospitalizations in same individual with bipolar disorder 2 years before and 2 years after starting clozapine (Nielson et al., 2012). A small number (1.5%) of adults with bipolar disorder were prescribed clozapine. On clozapine, patients had a significant decrease in the number of psychiatric hospital admissions (from a mean of 3.2 to 2.0) and a significant decrease in the number of days in hospital (from a mean of 177.8 to 34.6).

Clozapine has also been used in small open-label trials for treatment-resistant bipolar illness. Three notable such trials had inconsistent methods. Two (Calabrese et al., 1996; Suppes et al., 1999) included patients with schizoaffective disorder, while one did not (Green et al., 2000). Two (Calabrese et al., 1996; Green et al., 2000) used clozapine alone, while another (Suppes et al., 1999) added it to patients' current regimen. However, all three studies were consistent in that all found significant decreases in scores on the Brief Psychiatric Rating Scale (BPRS) (Overall & Gorham, 1962) and the Young Mania Rating Scale (Young et al., 1978) with clozapine treatment.

Clozapine is recommended for treatment of acute mania as a third-line agent in the Canadian Network for Mood and Anxiety Treatments (CANMAT) and the International Society for Bipolar Disorders (ISBD) 2018 guidelines for the management of patients with bipolar disorder (Yatham et al., 2018).

5.6.3 Severe borderline personality disorder

In Denmark, investigators (Rohde et al., 2018) reviewed nationwide records to identify all patients with BPD and a restricted subgroup comprising those without additional diagnoses of schizophrenia, schizoaffective disorder, or bipolar disorder, called the "BPD-specific patients." They compared the number of certain events 2 years before and 2 years after first filling a prescription for clozapine. After clozapine use, all BPD and BPD-specific patients had significantly fewer psychiatric hospitalizations and fewer days in hospital.

Severely ill patients with BPD can be treated in public hospitals where they often pose grave risks of suicide, self-injury, and assaults on staff and can require extraordinary levels of observation. Clozapine may benefit this group. When four women in a North Carolina state hospital were treated with clozapine for BPD (Zarzar & McEvoy, 2013), their self-injury, suicidality, aggression, and need for one-on-one observation resolved, and all could be discharged. In a survey of clinicians working in a secure hospital in the United Kingdom (Haw & Stubbs, 2011), clozapine was the most commonly prescribed drug for borderline patients. Treating psychiatrists reported it was the drug most likely to lead to major improvement.

An open trial of clozapine at 25–100 mg/day over 16 weeks for severe "psychotic-like" symptoms in 12 inpatients with BPD (Benedetti et al., 1998) found that BPRS total scores declined after 4 weeks by 54% on average, a statistically significant change. After 16 weeks, the number of suicide attempts and fights also decreased significantly. After 16 weeks, almost all patients were discharged.

The American Psychiatric Association Practice Guideline for the Treatment of Patients with Borderline Personality Disorder (Keepers et al., 2024) recommends treatment with a structured approach to psychotherapy. It does not support use of any one psychotropic medication, but suggests time-limited and targeted pharmacotherapy as an adjunctive to psychotherapy.

REFERENCES

Benedetti, F., Sforzini, L., Colombo, C., Maffei, C., & Smeraldi, E. (1998). Low-dose clozapine in acute and continuation treatment of severe borderline personality disorder. *Journal of Clinical Psychiatry* 59:103–107.

Calabrese, J. R., Kimmel, S. E., Woyshville, M. J., Rapport, D. J., Faust, C. J. Thompson, P. A., & Meltzer, H. Y. (1996). Clozapine for treatment-refractory mania. *American Journal of Psychiatry* 153(6):759–764.

Green, A. I., Tohen, M., Patel, J. K., Banov, M., DuRand, C., Berman, I., . . . & Schatzberg, A. F. (2000). Clozapine in the treatment of refractory psychotic mania. *American Journal of Psychiatry* 157(6):982–986.

Haw, C., & Stubbs, J. (2011). Medication for borderline personality disorder: A survey at a secure hospital. *International Journal of Psychiatry and Clinical Practice* 15(4):280–285.

Keepers, G. A., Fochtman, L. J., Anzia, J. M., Benjamin, S., Lyness, J. M., Mojtabai, R., . . . & Medicus, J. (2024). The American Psychiatric Association practice guideline for the treatment of patients with borderline personality disorder. *American Journal of Psychiatry* 181(11):1024–1028.

Lahteenvuo, M., Paljarvi, T., Tanskanen, A., Taipale, H., & Tiihonen, J. (2023). Real-world effectiveness of pharmacological treatments for bipolar disorder: Register-based national cohort study. *British Journal of Psychiatry* 223:456–464.

Nielsen, J., Kane, J. M., & Correll, C. U. (2012). Real-world effectiveness of clozapine in patients with bipolar disorder: Results from a 2-year mirror-image study. *Bipolar Disorders* 14(8):863–869.

Overall, J. E., & Gorham D. R. (1962). The Brief Psychiatric Rating Scale. *Psychological Reports* 10(3):799–812.

Rohde, C., Polcwiartek, C., Correll, C. U., & Nielsen, J. (2018). Real-world effectiveness of clozapine for borderline personality disorder: Results from a 2-year mirror-image study. *Journal of Personality Disorders* 32(6):823–837.

Suppes, T., Webb, A., Paul, B., Carmody, T. Kraemer, H., & Rush, A. J. (1999). Clinical outcome in a randomized 1-year trial of clozapine versus treatment as usual for patients with treatment-resistant illness and a history of mania. *American Journal of Psychiatry* 156(8):1164–1169.

Taipale, H., Lieslehto, J., Lahteenvuo, M., Hamina, A., Tanskanen, A., Mittendorfer-Rutz, E., . . . & Tiihonen, J. (2024). Real-world effectiveness of antidepressants, antipsychotics and their combinations in the maintenance treatment of psychotic depression: Evidence from within-subject analyses of two nationwide cohorts. *World Psychiatry* 23(2):276–284.

Yatham, L. N., Kennedy, S. H., Parikh, S. V., Schaffer, A., Bond, D. J., Frey, B. N., . . . & Berk, M. (2018). Canadian Network for Mood and Anxiety Treatments (CANMAT) and International Society for Bipolar Disorders (ISBD) 2018 guidelines for the management of patients with bipolar disorder. *Bipolar Disorders* 20(2):97–170.

Young, R. C., Biggs, J. T., Ziegler, V. E., & Meyer, D. A. (1978). A rating scale for mania: Reliability, validity and sensitivity. *British Journal of Psychiatry* 133:429–435.

Zarzar, T., & McEvoy, J. (2013). Clozapine for self-injurious behavior in individuals with borderline personality disorder. *Therapeutic Advances in Psychopharmacology* 3(5):272–274.

5.7 THE RIGHT TO ADEQUATE TREATMENT

5.7.1 "The Right to Treatment"

Morton Birnbaum, a physician and lawyer, wrote "The Right to Treatment" (1960), in which he argued that psychiatric patients with involuntary legal status have the right to adequate treatment, defined as restoration to health and freedom as soon as possible. Without adequate treatment, those held involuntarily are inmates held in mental prisons, not patients in hospitals. And without recognition of the right to treatment, states can understaff and underfund their hospitals and thereby limit psychiatrists' ability to offer more than custodial care.

Birnbaum recognized potential problems with mandating standards of care, including difficulties recruiting staff and the prohibitive expense to states. He suggested that public hospitals offer clinical staff salaries on par with what they could earn in private practice. He also suggested that the federal government financially support state hospitals.

Birnbaum was influential. The *Wyatt v. Stickney* (1971) decision on the right to treatment drew on the ideas and language of "The Right to Treatment."

5.7.2 *Wyatt v. Stickney*

When the state of Alabama terminated the employment of 99 staff members at Bryce Hospital in Tuscaloosa, the employees sued to be reinstated. They added a patient litigant, Ricky Wyatt, to also claim that patient treatment suffered as a result of the terminations.

In his 1971 *Wyatt v. Stickney* decision, Judge Johnson wrote that the state had a right to dismiss employees, but also that Bryce Hospital patients had a right to individual treatment that would give each a realistic chance of improvement in their condition, if not cure. Citing Alabama's expenditures for patient care, the least in the 50 states, Judge Johnson opined that the failure of Bryce Hospital to supply adequate treatment was due to lack of operating funds. (He also wrote that, of 5,000 patients 1,500–1,600 were geriatric and 1,000 had mental retardation and did not need psychiatric treatment.)

The state of Alabama had 6 months to fully implement adequate treatment and failed, so Judge Johnson mandated exacting standards for staffing and patient care. Birnbaum disagreed with the standards imposed because he believed they created enormous financial demands on states that would only lead to massive patient discharges. Fear of such standards caused states to do as Birnbaum predicted. Birnbaum's goal all along was improved treatment, not hospital closing (Mental Illness Policy Org, n.d.).

5.7.3 Comment

In our preceding cases, Mr. J., Mr. K., and Mr. L. all had a right to individual treatment that would give each a realistic opportunity to be cured or to improve their mental condition. They had a right to active, aggressive treatment, not custodial care. Their treatment required a trial of clozapine. Of the three, Mr. L. had the best response. Though none was cured, all had substantial benefit in improved functioning.

REFERENCES

Birnbaum, M. (1960). The right to treatment. *American Bar Association* 46(5):499–505.

Mental Illness Policy Org. (n.d.). Right to treatment: *Wyatt v. Stickney* – Case summary. Accessed on November 16, 2025, from: https://mentalillnesspolicy.org/legal/wyatt-stickney-right-treatment.html

Wyatt v. Stickney. 325 F. Supp. 781 (M.D. Ala. 1971).

6

MEDICATION OVER OBJECTION

This chapter reviews the history of legal thinking behind current laws concerning the patient who refuses treatment and details how those laws govern the process for obtaining a court order for treatment over objection. It includes two cases in which medication over objection was effective.

6.1 CASE M: A FLIRTATIOUS MAN

6.1.1 Case

Mr. M. was a man in his 20s who was admitted to a state psychiatric hospital after he was found not fit to stand trial for a misdemeanor charge involving a woman. His charges were dropped.

Interview

On admission, his female psychiatrist found a buoyant young man dressed in a tattered hoodie and flimsy sneakers. In this drab and unfamiliar setting, Mr. M. was pleased. He said he was very happy to see such a beautiful woman, leaned in close, and asked where she lived and if she was married. No, he never experienced hallucinations. No, he did not think of hurting himself or anyone else. Life was too sweet for such ideas! He had plans! He could already speak French and German and aimed to learn every other European language. He would get a job as an auto mechanic after he studied from a book.

Before the arrest, he was fine, he said, though worried about getting a job. Worry had caused him to sleep little, just 2 to 4 hours per night for the past 3 years, though he was not tired during the day. For 4 years he had been working double shifts as a handyman in an apartment building but quit the previous year because of a misunderstanding with a female tenant. While at work he would drink every day. Not a problem, he said, as long as he did not bother others. Though he had many family members in the area with whom he was welcome to live, he chose to live on the streets for a while, just for fun. This way, he could sleep when he wanted, get up when he wanted, be his own man. Before his arrest he had been living on the streets for several months.

Arrest led to his first psychiatric assessment. In jail, he refused medication because he thought he was allergic to it and because there was no need because he did not believe he had a psychiatric problem.

History

Mr. M. Senior, the young man's father, had noted changes which led him to conclude that his son was sick and needed help. Mr. M. had been a diligent college student and handyman who was shy and polite and asked for his father's advice. Over the previous 2 years he acted in ways that did not conform to his conservative upbringing, such as smoking marijuana, drinking, and talking openly about sexual matters. His temperament was different; he would sing and laugh to himself, then quickly turn angry and confrontational.

With time, his functioning deteriorated. Because female tenants accused him of making sexual overtures, he was fired. His father asked him to stay, but Mr. M. moved out of his home, then turned up erratically, smelly and dirty, asking for money or a place to stay.

When Mr. M. Senior visited his son in jail, he heard him make strange and concerning claims, such as that he talked with kings and with the US president. He told jail employees that his son needed help and asked that he get it. Now that Mr. M. was hospitalized, Mr. M. Senior was in favor of medication treatment over objection, if necessary, or in his food.

Course of treatment

Mr. M.'s psychiatrist immediately ordered antipsychotic medication at a low dose, and Mr. M. immediately refused. He did not agree that he had any kind of problem, especially not mental illness, not what his doctor told him he had, which was mania or bipolar disorder. The doctor explained how she believed he could benefit from medication in that he would get serious, get focused, and stay out of trouble. Mr. M. worried that the medication offered was unnatural and bad for his already not-so-good health. His doctor noted that his physical exam and routine lab testing were normal. She tried to reassure him, explaining possible adverse effects and that she would start with a low dose and keep a close eye on him.

Mr. M. was not convinced. He refused each dose offered. On the ward, he sometimes joined in therapeutic groups with other patients but more often paced the hallways. Women quickly learned to keep their distance.

His psychiatrist testified in court for retention and treatment over objection with long-acting injectable antipsychotics. In court, Mr. M. worked against himself, yelling angrily and speaking out of turn. Ward staff in attendance called for additional men to stand by, but he did not try to assault anyone when the presiding judge ordered retention and treatment over objection. He did not struggle when given a low-dose long-acting intramuscular antipsychotic.

By the next week, Mr. M. was able to sit in groups and pay attention when his psychiatrist discussed the benefits and side effects of medication. He asked many questions, some irrelevant, but many relevant. He complained of feeling weak, tired, and dizzy. Gradually, he became less intrusive, less silly, less free and easy, and women complained less about his wandering hands

By the following week, he agreed to take a mood stabilizer. He was prescribed the lowest possible doses of all medications because he still complained of dizziness and tiredness. Contrary to his complaints, he rarely slept during the day.

Mr. M. started showing an interest in employment and housing after discharge. Eventually he agreed to return to his father's home. On the day of discharge, Mr. M. had an appointment at a state outpatient clinic. He said that he felt very well and that the medication he took helped him become less nervous. Though he was urged to continue taking it and warned of the risk of relapse, he was clear that he might discontinue. He said, "If at some point I think I am fine, I will not take it."

6.2 HOW TO OBTAIN A COURT ORDER FOR TREATMENT

Before resorting to a court hearing, Mr. M.'s psychiatrist was obliged to work to obtain his voluntary cooperation, explain the risks and benefits of treatment, and tell him about any alternative options. But her patient lacked the capacity to make a decision based on facts. He did not agree that he had a mental illness; he was happy just as he was. What he thought were risks of treatment, that is, side effects, were not. The benefits of treatment were many: foremost was that he could get his life back on track (i.e., return to employment, stop sleeping in a park, and stop getting arrested).

In court, Mr. M's psychiatrist had to make a convincing argument that he lacked capacity to make a reasoned decision about his treatment and that, for this particular man, the benefits of medication outweighed the risks (Behnke et al., 2003). Although not required by law, his doctor asserted that his illness caused what could be seen as dangerous behavior, as evidenced by his arrest.

Mr. M. recognized some benefit—that he was less nervous—but acknowledged that he might not continue treatment. The court order was limited to the hospital where he was treated, so he was free to stop taking medication as soon as he was discharged.

REFERENCE

Behnke, S. J., Pelin, M. L., & Bernstein, M. (2003). *The Essentials of New York Mental Health Law: A Straightforward Guide for Clinicians of All Disciplines*. New York: Norton.

6.3 THE RIGHT TO REFUSE TREATMENT

Before the late 1970s, state laws required patients' consent to medical treatment but not to psychiatric treatment. Psychiatric patients were an exception because they were considered incompetent to consent to or refuse treatment. The right to treat was considered inextricable from the right to commit, which was based on needing treatment. Thus, involuntary patients had no right to refuse. However, by 1971, being a proper subject for treatment was not a criteria for commitment in Massachusetts; dangerousness was (Appelbaum, 1994).

Rubie Rogers was a patient at Boston State Hospital who had been administered haloperidol against her will and, as a result, developed tardive dyskinesia. In 1975, attorneys brought suit in federal court on behalf of Ms. Rogers and other patients at the same hospital, challenging physicians' right to force patients to accept medications such as haloperidol (Appelbaum, 1994).

In 1979, Judge Tauro ruled that while the hospital had a duty to offer treatment, it did not have the right to impose treatment the patient refused. He forbade hospital staff to forcibly medicate voluntary or involuntary patients, except in emergency circumstances—that is, when failing to do so would bring about a substantial likelihood of physical harm to the patient or others. Tauro wrote that patients had the right to be left alone without "mind-altering" forced medications, medications that bring about "mind control" and impede their First Amendment right to generate ideas (*Rogers v. Okin*, 1979). His opinion rested heavily on the risks of adverse medication effects but barely mentioned therapeutic effects.

The case was litigated in other courts, and, finally, in 1983 (*Rogers v. Commissioner, Department of Mental Health*), the Massachusetts high court decided that competent patients have the right to refuse medication, but patients who are not competent do not. In nonemergent situations in the state of Massachusetts, a judge must find a patient not competent to decide to accept or reject medication and then issue a court order before medication can be administered over objection.

As a result of this and other right-to-refuse-treatment rulings, all states decided that voluntary patients have the right to refuse treatment. Massachusetts and the state in which Mr. M., the flirtatious man in our preceding case, was treated, adopted an approach in keeping with the Rogers decision, in which involuntary patients have the right to refuse unless a judge agrees that they are not competent and that treatment is appropriate (Appelbaum, 1994).

Other states adopted a different approach, one that does not require judicial review but does require procedures to ensure that treatment over objection for incompetent patients meets professional standards of care (Appelbaum, 1988). State laws can change with time.

REFERENCES

Appelbaum, P. S. (1988). The right to refuse treatment with antipsychotic medications: Retrospect and prospect. *American Journal of Psychiatry* 145(4):413–419.

Appelbaum, P. S. (1994). Right to refuse treatment with medication. In *Almost a Revolution: Mental Health Law and the Limits of Change*, pp. 114–162. New York: Oxford University Press.

Rogers v. Commissioner, Department of Mental Health. 458 N.E.2d 308 (Mass. 1983).
Rogers v. Okin. 478 F. Supp. 1342 (D. Mass. 1979).

6.4 CASE N: LOST A SON

6.4.1 Case

Mr. N. was a man in his 30s who was admitted to a state psychiatric hospital after being found not fit to stand trial on misdemeanor charges involving threats to his former high school teacher.

Interview

His psychiatrist found a neatly dressed man who was indignant that he was being asked to participate in a psychiatric exam. Straight away he declared he had no psychiatric problems and would take no medication. "You are violating the mental hygiene laws," he asserted, and he invited the psychiatrist to read over the statutes with him so the doctor could better understand them. He did not answer questions about allergies or alcohol and illicit drug use. When asked if he ever heard voices when no one was around, he answered, "Absolutely not!" Had he ever had thoughts of hurting himself? "Absolutely not!"

History

Mr. N. provided little information but much came with him. In addition to the required reports from the psychiatrists who determined he was unfit to stand trial, he came with letters from his former high school teacher and from his father pleading to have him held against his will in the hospital for long-term treatment.

His father had noticed trouble for years. After he graduated high school, he took jobs that never lasted. He complained that his coworkers talked about him and spied on him. Coworkers and bosses, like teachers and fellow students before them, all turned out to be incompetents. His son had been strange and distant, difficult to talk to and belligerent. Mr. N. confided that he was followed by agents of the CIA and that someone had entered his rented room and implanted something in his brain. His father heard him talking loudly to himself when he thought he was alone. He did not see any indication that he was using illicit drugs.

Mr. N. had resisted his father's efforts to get him into treatment, dodging inpatient psychiatric care twice. After admission to a general hospital psychiatric unit, he walked out abruptly and prematurely. Again, earlier in the year of his current admission, he agreed to inpatient treatment after his father bailed him out of jail, but signed himself out.

Course of treatment

On the ward Mr. N. refused to attend groups, refused a physical exam, refused to give a medical history, and refused routine admission lab testing. He refused every dose of antipsychotic medication nurses offered him. Instead, he spent his time in the dayroom watching TV or reading.

With ward staff, he argued and claimed he was abused. With his psychiatrist, he demanded a thicker, more comfortable mattress and insisted it could be provided to him when it could not. With other patients, he was disdainful. Other men who shared his room complained that he kept them up at night talking loudly to himself.

His psychiatrist applied for antipsychotic treatment over objection to treat his schizophrenia. Three weeks into his stay, with his father present, Mr. N. appeared in court for a hearing. Acting as his own lawyer, he argued with the judge, who often told him to stop talking. The judge signed an order allowing administration of an injectable long-acting antipsychotic every 2 weeks.

A week after his first injection, he still abhorred therapeutic groups but spent his time napping, reading, or playing cards with other patients and staff. He seemed more sociable and less intense, but, after 3 weeks, his father reported that Mr. N. told him that he was persecuted by hospital staff and given a second-rate mattress out of spite.

Five weeks after his first injection, he joined groups regularly, allowed blood and urine testing, and no longer kept his roommates up at night talking to himself. While he had become much less hostile and haughty, he maintained he did not need medication and would not take it willingly.

A few weeks later, Mr. N. was engaged in his work in the print shop and not in arguments about his mattress. He agreed with his doctor that he was more relaxed but believed it was because he had become accustomed to the hospital, not because of medication. Together with his social worker, he completed a Social Security application so he would have an income. His treatment team offered discharge to a supervised residence and vocational training, but his father weighed in with his preference that his son stay hospitalized until he could accept that he had a mental illness.

Mr. N. accepted a clinic appointment and a bed in a transitional residence, knowing that staff there would help him meet his goals, which were a more permanent place to live and a job. While he refused to believe he had a mental illness, he said he would take medication if his doctor advised it.

A few weeks later, Mr. N. Senior called for news. He had heard nothing from his son. Mr. N.'s psychiatrist called the clinic to pass on his father's request and reached a clinician who was working with Mr. N. Mr. N. wanted no contact, she said, so she would not share information with his father. She knew that, as an adult, Mr. N. had the right to make this decision.

6.4.2 Comment

That Mr. N. agreed to take medication was cause for hope, but without court-mandated outpatient treatment, for which he was not eligible, he could stop medication at any time. His father wanted him to be hospitalized until he agreed he had a mental illness, but he could not be held involuntarily for that purpose alone. He no longer met criteria for involuntary hospital retention and had a right to be treated in the least restrictive setting (see Chapters 10.1 and 10.3).

His father wanted a recovered son, but also one who would agree he had a mental illness, appreciate his efforts to help him, and continue their relationship. He did not. A job and a relationship with clinicians in a clinic and with staff in a residence could hold him in treatment. With time, continued treatment could possibly help him reconcile with his family.

7

PATIENTS WITH INTENSIVE NURSING NEEDS

This chapter describes the care and treatment of two men with chronic, debilitating neurologic disorders. Both were admitted to and retained in a state hospital on a forensic legal status. The chapter explains their legal status and others, including not fit to stand trial and not guilty by reason of insanity.

7.1 CASE O: A MAN WITH HUNTINGTON'S DISEASE

7.1.1 Case

Mr. O. was a man in his mid-50s who was admitted to a state psychiatric hospital after being charged with a nonviolent felony and found not fit to stand trial. His charges were not dropped, so the hospital was responsible for restoring his fitness to enable him to stand trial.

Interview

On first interview, his psychiatrist met a lanky man with an intent gaze whose body was in constant motion. A shoulder shrugged, his neck twisted, his trunk thrust out. When asked a question, he would pause, summon an effort, and produce a short, concise response. When asked, "How are you?" he replied, "Good. And you?" He lurched and teetered his way around the ward holding onto a walker, causing anyone near to worry that he would soon topple over. (The walker was soon replaced by a wheelchair.)

History

Fitness examiners wrote that while he had no psychotic symptoms, he had cognitive problems. For example, he was off by more than 10 years in naming the year, and he struggled with recalling numbers and simple arithmetic. A psychiatrist examiner wrote that Mr. O. had trouble walking, but the doctor attributed this and his memory impairments to a head injury he suffered 10 years earlier. A second examiner noted involuntary movements and mildly impaired speech articulation, without speculating on their etiology. Mr. O. told fitness examiners he had never been in psychiatric or substance abuse treatment. He had not worked in 10 years and collected social security for a medical, not a neurologic or psychiatric, disability. Just prior to his arrest he lived alone in a rented room.

A nurse working in the jail where he was held prior to state hospital transfer described jerky uncontrollable movements and also ascribed them to past head injury. The nurse added that he needed a cane to walk and had a recent weight loss of 30–40 lbs.

A search undertaken at the state hospital for records of previous hospitalizations yielded only one, from a community hospital where he had been admitted for a fall more than a year before he was admitted to the state hospital. Doctors at the hospital wrote he had a history of a choreiform movement disorder that they left unnamed.

Course of treatment

Mr. O. demonstrated impaired balance, gait, and posture; muscle rigidity; and trouble swallowing and speaking. He could control his bladder and feed himself. A psychiatrist who was also trained as a neurologist took one look and said he had Huntington's disease. It took months of cajoling but finally, accompanied by a trusted nurse, Mr. O. traveled to a local general hospital and allowed genetic testing, which confirmed the doctor's opinion. He and Woodie Guthrie had the same disease, an unrelenting, progressive, neurodegenerative disease of genetic origin. Because the gene is autosomal dominant, his children had a 50% chance of inheriting his illness (Ghosh & Tabrizi, 2018).

Mr. O. was treated on a special unit in the hospital for patients with greater than average medical and nursing needs. Despite his persistent and laborious efforts and those of his treatment team, he could not accomplish the learning he needed to become fit to stand trial. A psychologist completed cognitive testing that showed that, despite genuine effort, Mr. O. demonstrated poor memory, poor attention, and limited ability to learn a new task.

Mr. O. had his own ideas about what he could do. His plan was to get a cane to help him walk and return to his home. He told anyone who would listen, "Don't forget about me. Home today."

The treatment team had no family contact. When asked for a phone number, Mr. O. would offer a string of digits, his best guess for his mother's phone number, but again and again the numbers connected to nobody. Finally he recalled his mother's name, a town, and a street. An internet search produced a full address to which his ward social worker sent a letter. Weeks later, when the letter was nearly forgotten, she got a call. Her patient's mother was seriously ill, but Mr. O's brother found and opened the letter. Mr. O. was found by his family. His brother became a regular conduit to his family as the social worker called regularly, informing him of Mr. O's illness and treatment and of his family's risk.

One day during lunch, Mr. O. choked. An attendant performed the Heimlich maneuver, and internists and nurses rushed to attend to him. After a 3-week stay in a local hospital for aspiration pneumonia, he returned to the state hospital where he immediately pulled out his nasal cannula. When asked about his mood, he said, "Good." But he was not so good; his condition had deteriorated. Unable to control his bladder, he needed diapers. He needed help moving from bed to chair, more help bathing and dressing. Attendants had to spoon-feed him.

Soon after he returned from the general hospital, he was found with a blanket over his head. "I want to go home," he said, "I want to be left alone." He hated that he could not care for himself. Attendants knew this and allowed him to do all he could. He hated most soft foods and being fed. After two spoonsful he rejected what was offered and asked for peanut butter and jelly, cereal, a hamburger, or "chicken that looks like chicken."

A few weeks after he returned from the community hospital, he was approached by his ward internist about a Do Not Resuscitate (DNR) order. She asked, "How are you?" And he replied, "OK. How are you?" She described chest compressions and intubation. He did not want either.

"What does that mean?" the internist asked.

"I would die," he said.

"Why would you want to die?"

"I feel old and sick."

Mr. O. could not understand or remember the information necessary to demonstrate fitness to stand trial. No amount of coaching could overcome his impairments. Therefore, his charges were eventually dropped; he was "Jacksoned," referring to *Jackson v. Indiana*, a United States Supreme Court decision of 1972. His legal status was changed from forensic to civil. A nursing home would not accept him as a forensic patient with active criminal charges, but, once his charges were dropped, he could be referred.

REFERENCES

Ghosh, R., & Tabrizi, S. J. (2018). Clinical features of Huntington's disease. *Advances in Experimental Medicine and Biology* 1049:1–28

Jackson v. Indiana. 406 U.S. 715 (1972), 113.

7.2 TYPES OF FORENSIC LEGAL STATUS

7.2.1 Not fit to stand trial or incompetent to stand trial

All defendants in the United States have the right to understand and participate in their own legal defense and court proceedings. Criteria for fitness or competence as delineated in the *Dusky v. United States* (1960) Supreme Court decision are having a sufficient present ability to consult with a defense attorney with a reasonable degree of rational understanding, and a rational as well as factual understanding of the proceedings.

When defendants assessed for competence to stand trial are found lacking, they can be referred for restoration of competence, a process that involves both psychiatric treatment and instruction on the court process (Wik et al., 2020). Assessment and restoration are separate processes that can take place in separate locations. Where and how these processes unfold varies by state and time, but restoration has most often occurred in state hospitals (Murrie et al., 2022).

Between 2005 and 2014, state hospitals in all states plus the District of Columbia experienced an increase in the numbers of patients who were found incompetent to stand trial (Wik et al., 2020). Increased demand spurred new laws and practices. As of 2016, 16 states had at least one outpatient restoration program—some in jail, others in community clinics (Murrie et al., 2022).

State laws can distinguish between defendants charged with misdemeanors and those charged with felonies. The majority of states hospitalize most, if not all, people charged with felonies who require competency restoration, while a few states do not typically admit people charged with misdemeanors for competency restoration services (Wik et al., 2017, p. 47). In the state where Mr. N., Mr. O., and others in this book were treated, when defendants are charged with a misdemeanor, charges are dropped and the person is committed to an appropriate institution for care and treatment (New York State Office of Mental Health, n.d.).

7.2.2 *Jackson v. Indiana* and its results

Theon Jackson was 27 years old, deaf and mute, with minimal education and minimal ability to sign when, in May of 1968, he was charged in the state of Indiana with two robberies. Fitness examiners opined that he was not fit to stand trial due to his "mental deficiency" and "communication defect." Although these conditions were considered permanent, he was committed to a state hospital until he could become fit.

In 1969, his attorney filed for a new trial, arguing that Mr. Jackson could not be restored to competency and therefore was committed for life. His case was appealed to the Supreme Court, which, in June of 1972, decided that Mr. Jackson's commitment violated his constitutional rights (Parker, 2011). The Court ruled that a person hospitalized for fitness restoration cannot be held "more than the reasonable period of time necessary" to determine if that person is likely to become fit in the foreseeable future (*Jackson v. Indiana*, 1972).

The phrase "reasonable period of time" is vague and interpreted differently in different states. In New York state, a felony defendant can be held involuntarily on a commitment to restore fitness for up to two-thirds of the maximum sentence the patient would have received if convicted (New York State Office of Mental Health, n.d.). In Texas (Code of Criminal Procedure, n.d.), a felony defendant may be committed to treatment for competency restoration for as long as the maximum sentence the individual would have received if convicted, but not longer. Patients who can no longer be held for fitness restoration may be committed to a psychiatric hospital on a civil status.

Theo Jackson was ordered released from an Indiana state hospital in September 1972, with final diagnosis of deaf-mutism. By this time, his functioning in the hospital and extensive cognitive testing demonstrated that he did not have intellectual impairment (Parker, 2011).

7.2.3 Not guilty by reason of insanity

The legal standard for the insanity defense has been controversial and has varied over time and between states. The Insanity Defense Reform Act of 1984 states that, in a federal prosecution, the insanity defense is an affirmative defense that, at the time of the offense, the defendant, as a result of mental disease or defect, was unable to appreciate the nature and quality or the wrongfulness of his or her acts (Comprehensive Crime Control Act, 1984).

Although they attract much attention, insanity defense cases have been rare. On average in the United States, the insanity defense has been raised in fewer than 1% of all felony cases and has been successful in about 15–28% of those (Borum & Fulero, 1999). In the state hospitals of 31 states that provided data, numbers of patients found not guilty by reason of insanity or guilty but mentally ill increased minimally from 1999 to 2014 (Wik et al., 2017).

It could be that defense attorneys warn their clients that, if an insanity defense is successful, they would be held in hospital indefinitely, until no longer mentally ill and no longer dangerous, as decided by the *Jones v. U.S.* Supreme Court decision (1983). Unless accused of a very serious crime, the defendant could spend more time in psychiatric hospitals than he or she would in prison if found guilty.

REFERENCES

Borum, R., & Fulero, S. M. (1999). Empirical research on the insanity defense and attempted reforms: evidence toward informed policy. *Law and Human Behavior* 23(3):375–394.

Code of Criminal Procedure (n.d.). Title 1: Code of Criminal Procedure. Chapter 46B. Incompetency to Stand Trial. Subchapter A. General provisions. Accessed on November 17, 2025, from: https://statutes.capitol.texas.gov/docs/CR/htm/CR.46B.htm

Comprehensive Crime Control Act of 1984. (1984). Title IV (Pub. L. 98–473, S. 1762, 98 Stat. 1976. Accessed on November 17, 2025, from: https://www.congress.gov/bill/98th-congress/senate-bill/1762

Dusky v. United States. 362 U. S. 402 (1960).

Jackson v. Indiana. 406 U. S. 715 (1972).

Jones v. United States. 463 U. S. 354 (1983).

Murrie, D. C., Gowensmith, W. N., Kois, L. E., & Packer, I. K. (2023). Evaluations of competence to stand trial are evolving amid a national "competency crisis." *Behavioral Sciences & the Law* 41(5):310–325.

New York State Office of Mental Health. (n.d.). Populations served in OMH forensic facilities. Accessed on November 17, 2025, from: https://omh.ny.gov/omhweb/forensic/populations_served.htm

Parker, G. F. (2011). An historical review of the legal and personal background to *Jackson v. Indiana. Journal of the American Academy of Psychiatry and the Law* 39: 86–92.

Wik, A., Hollen, V., & Fisher, W. H. (2017). Forensic patients in state psychiatric hospitals. National Association of State Mental Health Program Directors publication. Accessed on November 17, 2025, from: https://www.nri-inc.org/media/1318/tac-paper-9-forensic-patients-in-state-hospitals-final-09-05-2017.pdf

Wik, A., Hollen, V., & Fisher, W. H. (2020). Forensic patients in state psychiatric hospitals 1999–2016. *CNS Spectrums* 25(2):196–206.

7.3 CASE P: A MAN WITH PARKINSON'S DISEASE

7.3.1 Case

Mr. P. was a man in his 70s who was found not fit to stand trial on charges of a felony sexual offense; he was sent to a state psychiatric hospital for treatment to restore his competency.

Interview

His psychiatrist found Mr. P. reclining in a geriatric (geri) chair. He smiled, nodded, said he felt fine and then asked, "Where am I?"

Psychiatrist: In a hospital. Do you know why you're in a hospital?
Mr. P.: Because I have an illness.
Psychiatrist: What illness?
Mr. P.: None.
Psychiatrist: Is it a physical or mental illness?
Mr. P.: Mental.
Psychiatrist: What kind?

Mr. P. couldn't explain. He denied that he was depressed, confused, heard voices, or felt anxious. When the doctor asked again about his mental illness, he replied he had a physical illness. What kind of physical illness? He wasn't sure.

When the psychiatrist asked if he had lived in a nursing home, he allowed that he had, but just for a bit, then he twisted in his chair and complained of leg pain where he was bruised. After he admitted that he fell, his doctor told him to ask staff to help him so he wouldn't have accidents. Mr. P. couldn't say why he had lived in a nursing home or much about his past. He related that he had moved to the state where he was living 12 years previously, when he was age 10.

History

At the state hospital, a social worker contacted his Adult Protective Services guardian, who had first met Mr. P. about 6 years earlier when her agency started providing home care services in his apartment. On first entering his apartment, workers were greeted by hoards of roaches and the stench of urine. The apartment resembled a sailing ship with ropes hanging from the ceilings for Mr. P. to grab for balance when he walked. The guardian found papers in the apartment that revealed that Mr. P. had a college degree and a professional license, but she found no leads to family members: no names, no phone numbers, no photos. Letters she mailed to return addresses from holiday cards brought no replies.

About 4 years before he was admitted to the state hospital, Mr. P. was placed in a nursing home because he was found lying on the floor of his apartment in a puddle of urine. He had fallen and lay there for 2 days. The guardian related that administrators at the home tried transferring him to many, many other places, but none would take him. Administrators believed his inappropriate actions were "behavioral", meaning he was able to control himself, but chose not to, and in this way justified their use of the criminal justice system. They encouraged the family of a woman he had allegedly groped to press charges.

Records sent from that facility to the state hospital did not note any family contacts, where he had lived, who brought him to their facility or why, or when he had developed Parkinson's disease. They did contain numerous complaints about his behavior, particularly that he hid food and sexually assaulted female residents.

The allegation of groping led to the first arrest of his life and to incarceration in a jail unit for medically frail inmates. There he awaited the outcome of his case, which was, after several months, a sentence to time served. Mr. P. returned to the nursing home but was soon arrested again for another alleged groping incident; he was returned to the same unit.

Staff at the jail unit struggled to meet Mr. P.'s nursing and medical needs. He fell out of his wheelchair. He choked on his food and so required a pureed diet and supervision when he ate. He could not cooperate with his care and had no idea why he was locked up. "It must a mistake," he told a physical therapist.

Forensic examiners noted that he had been diagnosed with Parkinson's disease. He did not know his charges, the date, or his age. He was found not fit to stand trial, and he was transferred from jail to a state hospital.

Course of treatment

Mr. P. kept on falling. He could not lie still in his chair but instead would climb out, try to walk, topple over, and then crawl to the ward door to get out and go home. Attendants had to watch him constantly. He would sleep until mid-afternoon, then resume his efforts to walk or crawl to the exit and escape. After a few days and some medication adjustments he could sleep at night, and during the day he watched TV and joined groups of patients in activities such as in-chair exercise. Throughout the day he reclined in front of a TV with an attendant beside him. His female nurse said he was a little "hand happy," by which she meant his hands would wander when she took his vital signs, but he would stop when caught.

Mr. P. never became fit and never returned to the nursing home, but died at a local community hospital due to an acute infectious illness.

7.3.2 Comment

When family cannot take up the burden, it falls on the community to care for disabled citizens. Mr. P. was without family to care or advocate for him, and he was clearly disabled. But what institution, what group would be the caretaker? Institutions can be motivated to pass along burdensome or dangerous patients to somewhere else. Mr. O. and Mr. P. required constant attention and intensive nursing and medical supervision.

Nursing homes typically care for and supervise residents with chronic disabling neurologic illness that can be associated with behavior problems. In Mr. P.'s case, Parkinson's disease and its treatment are associated with disordered impulse control (Weintraub & Claassen, 2017). The home that expelled Mr. P. used the criminal justice system to pass him along. Both the jail and the state hospital were legally required to accept him.

REFERENCE

Weintraub, D., & Claassen, D. O. (2017). Impulse control and related disorders in Parkinson's disease. *International Review of Neurobiology* 133:679–717.

SECTION II

Discharge Planning

8

DISCHARGE TO FAMILY

This chapter shows how treatment teams work as partners with families to support patients after discharge. By means of four cases, it gives examples of family conflicts and responsibilities that result from having a seriously mentally ill family member. Short discussions consider motherhood in public hospital patients and employment in adults with bipolar disorder. A longer discussion reviews studies on the association of childhood maltreatment with adult psychiatric problems.

8.1 CASE Q: DISCHARGE OF A MOTHER

8.1.1 Case

Ms. Q. was a woman in her 30s who was admitted to a state psychiatric hospital in July after she was found not fit to stand trial on misdemeanor charges. Her charges were dropped.

Interview

Ms. Q. looked around the admitting office and commented on the appearance of the nurse, the therapy aide, the safety officer, and the bare walls. She herself was unkempt and unadorned, her tee-shirt stained and her hair shorn willy-nilly.

Her doctor asked how she was feeling. "I'm feeling good! Better than usual! I feel good all the time!" she replied. She tore into her lunch of a cold and solidified portion of tuna noodle casserole with diced carrots, a slice of bread in a cellophane bag, a carton of milk, and a small tub of apple juice.

Ms. Q. was scattered, without the ability to concentrate enough to recall three objects or repeat a series of numbers. It hurt her brain, she said. She wasn't loud but had a lot to say. Any question set her off on a ramble, from which her psychiatrist roped her in to get a relevant answer. What was going on in the news? "Madness. Shooting and killing," she said. She denied hearing voices others did not and emphatically denied wanting to die. In her meanderings, she confided that she could see through people and wanted to be in the hospital to share her love. She also volunteered that people got angry with her sometimes because she talked too much.

She said she had been taking medications; she needed them, they helped her sleep and control her emotional problems, problems she had had since she was a teenager.

History

Her clinic psychiatrist told her inpatient psychiatrist that Ms. Q. had been doing well; this was her first hospitalization in years. Neither he nor the clinic social worker knew that she cared for her toddler in a small apartment without nearby family to readily check in on them. Her mother said that every 3 months her daughter had been seeing her psychiatrist and getting a prescription for her regular daily medication. She last saw her psychiatrist in February. In May, she appeared for her clinic appointment, but the doctor did not. Ms. Q. went home, did not return to the clinic, and ran out of medication. Within a few weeks, she was arrested. Both her mother and her clinic psychiatrist confirmed that she did not drink to excess or use illicit drugs.

Course of treatment

Ms. Q. spent much of her days pacing the hallways and talking to herself. "Just talking to myself," she said, "I don't hear voices." Several times a day she changed her clothes or restyled her hair. In groups, she had a hard time paying attention but made a whole-hearted effort, and, in some, she took notes. Other patients complained that she tried to engage them in long, unwelcome conversations. A female patient complained in a community meeting that an unnamed but easily identified chatterbox in her dorm kept her awake at night, and she threatened to smack that chatterbox if she didn't shut up. The chatterbox confided that she was hyper and wanted to be less so. She asked for medication.

By her fourth week in hospital, Ms. Q. had given up pacing the halls and her constant talking and instead sat in the dayroom engrossed in the local newspaper. She could sit in one place for 45 minutes or more, and she wore the same clothes all day. Now a worried mother, she listened attentively and questioned closely as she and her psychiatrist met with the ward social worker to discuss plans for her child and herself.

By this time, Ms. Q's mother had given up her daughter's apartment because there was no money for the rent. After 30 days in jail, Ms. Q.'s benefits checks stopped. The social worker offered Ms. Q. a few options, but she chose to take her child from her mother's care and join her sister and her sister's children in their already crowded apartment—temporarily—as her mother began the search for another apartment. And so, on the morning of the appointed day, she packed up her clothing, brushes, and hair extensions and said goodbye.

8.1.2 Comment

Ms. Q. and her family were the victims of poor continuity of care. She knew she needed medication and was willing to take it. Outpatient treatment worked for her until no doctor showed up to renew her lithium prescription. No one from the clinic, and neither Ms. Q. nor her family, called to reschedule.

8.1.3 Notes on seriously mentally ill women as mothers

Two surveys of female state hospital patients determined how many were mothers. Of 52 women in one facility (Joseph et al., 1999), 61.5% had at least one child. Only 22% had seen their children in the past week, and 38% had not seen them in more than 2 years. Twenty-one percent had full custody. Nearly all mothers of young children said it was very important to them to help raise their children. Patient diagnoses were not noted.

In another state hospital (Benders-Hadi et al., 2013), 50 of 130 women or 38.5% were mothers. Of these, 45.8% had at least weekly contact with their children, and 54.2% reported they were primary caretakers. Patients said that motherhood gave purpose to their lives and helped them stay in treatment. Nearly 80% of the mothers were diagnosed with schizophrenia or schizoaffective disorder.

Other investigators (Miller & Finnerty, 1996) compared 46 women with schizophrenic disorders to 50 women with medical problems. Both groups of women were treated at the same medical center. The two groups were not different in number of pregnancies, but the mentally ill group were significantly more likely to have had abortions. Women with schizophrenia were significantly more likely to have lost custody of their children, but most of those who had custody felt strongly involved with their role as mothers and wanted to maintain custody.

REFERENCES

Benders-Hadi, N., Barber, M., & Alexander, M. J. (2013). Motherhood in women with serious mental illness. *Psychiatric Quarterly* 84:65–72.

Joseph, J. G., Joshi, S. V., Lewin, A. B., & Abrams, M. (1999). Characteristics and perceived needs of mothers with serious mental illness. *Psychiatric Services* 50(10):1357–1359.

Miller, L. J., & Finnerty, M. (1996). Sexuality, pregnancy, and childbearing among women with schizophrenia-spectrum disorders. *Psychiatric Services* 47(5):502–506.

8.2 CASE R: DISCHARGE OF A HUSBAND AND FATHER

8.2.1 Case

Mr. R. was a man in his 40s who was admitted to a state psychiatric hospital after being found not fit to stand trial on misdemeanor charges. His charges were dropped before he was admitted.

Interview

Sitting for his first interview, Mr. R. was giddy. He laughed readily, talked excitedly, and sat a little too close. He told his psychiatrist that his current manic episode started when he noticed strange changes in his body, decided that these changes were due to his medication, and so stopped taking it. Five or six weeks later, it happened again. He got manic. At the height of the pressure and confusion of his manic episode, he was arrested.

He said that this was the seventh time in 20 years he had become manic, the third time in 4 years. Each time it was the same: he got a lot sharper, stopped his medication, then got hyper and stopped eating. Then heavy-duty paranoia set in. The television and strangers on the street talked about him. He felt surrounded and watched. Buildings took ominous shapes. Finally, he restarted medication, and it brought him back to earth.

Before his illness, Mr. R. graduated from college and held white-collar employment, first in larger then in smaller companies. But for more than 10 years he had not worked and instead collected Social Security disability checks. He could not recall ever getting depressed.

Course of treatment

Mrs. R. spoke with her husband's psychiatrist soon after he was admitted. She and Mr. R. had been married for more than 20 years, but separated for 2 years. "Almost all those years, he was sick," she said, "but he was OK when he took his medicine. Sometimes he believed he would be all right without it and stopped, like last year when he had to be admitted to a local hospital." Before last year, he'd gone a few years without getting sick. When he was not taking his medication, he got overexcited about things, loud, insistent, and in your face. When she believed he wasn't taking medication and told him so, he turned angry, complaining it made him sluggish and heavy.

By the time of his current admission, Mrs. R. had lost patience with her husband. She wanted him to get more of a life, a life more apart from hers, and more productive. He picked up their children from after-school activities but otherwise just sat around at his house, watching sports on television. He had no interests besides his wife and kids. She wanted him to work, to contribute more to the support of the children. He wouldn't. He was afraid of losing his benefits. For years, she told him that he could work and make a little money and still get Social Security Disability (SSD) payments (for disabled adults who have a significant work history), but he argued and never did. She wanted a divorce and knew he did not.

The next week, Mrs. R. called to complain that Mr. R. called her frequently imploring her not to divorce him. He confessed that he called twice a day, at least. His wife and the kids were his life, and he told her so.

On the ward, Mr. R. could not stop talking. In his constant arguments with his psychiatrist, he could not believe talkativeness was a symptom of his illness. This was just who he was. He had always been a motormouth, even as a child. He organized the other patients to sign a petition requesting more sports channels on television. In group discussions, he entertained his fellow patients with stories of his daring adventures when he was manic.

After a few weeks, he confided that he believed his wife had another man in her life. She wanted him to sign divorce papers. He had to say to her, "Well, not 'you win,' but OK." His wife said that Mr. R. was calmer when he called, which was about every other day. He had given up pressuring her to continue their relationship and to drop her plan to divorce. He called his children every day.

His reorganized medication regimen was working. The TV still talked about him, but rarely. He was singing in the morning and sleeping well at night. His waist had grown thicker, but, if he noticed, he said nothing. Before he left the hospital to live near his children, Mr. R. wanted to know how he could remember to take his medication and how he could work. He was discharged on lithium, divalproex, and risperidone.

8.2.2 Notes on employment, Social Security, rehabilitation

Approximately 40–60% of people in the United States with established bipolar illness are employed (Marwaha et al., 2013). However, many (30–40% in one review) have difficulties functioning at work (Marwaha et al., 2013), and most miss time at work due to psychiatric problems (Zimmerman et al., 2010). People with multiple hospital admissions for bipolar illness, like Mr. R., are less likely to be working than those with only one admission (Dion et al., 1988). Those who remain employed often transition over time to jobs that are less demanding or jobs of lower status (Marwaha et al., 2013).

Mrs. R. complained that her husband chose not to work and make a little money because he feared losing his SSD benefits. Social Security Administration guidelines change over time. In 2025 (Social Security Administration, 2025) people on SSD could continue benefits and work within limits. They were allowed a 9-month trial period when they could work and still receive full benefits. The beneficiary had to earn more than $1,160 in a month for that month to count as 1 of the 9 months. After the 9-month trial period, benefits could continue for any month in which the beneficiary did not earn more than $1,620 per month.

As an outpatient, Mr. R. got medication that alleviated his symptoms, but he needed more. He needed psychosocial rehabilitation, a broad category of services to support the functioning of people with psychiatric problems. Services can include housing and supervision, but also what Mr. R. needed: help understanding his benefits and a job program, such as supported employment, to get back into the workforce. Research suggests that 40–60% of patients enrolled in supported employment obtain employment, compared to 20% of similar patients not enrolled in supported employment (Bond, 2004).

REFERENCES

Bond, G. R. (2004). Supported employment: Evidence for a evidence-based practice. *Psychiatric Rehabilitation Journal* 27:345–359.

Dion, G. L., Tohen, M., Anthony, W. A., & Waternaux, C. S. (1988). Symptoms and functioning of patients with bipolar disorder six months after hospitalization. *Hospital and Community Psychiatry* 39:652–657.

Marwaha, S., Durrani, A., & Singh, S. (2013). Employment outcomes in people with bipolar disorder: A systematic review. *Acta Psychiatrica Scandinavica* 128:179–193.

Social Security Administration. (2025). Working while disabled: How we can help. Accessed October 10, 2025, from: https://www.ssa.gov/pubs/EN-05-10095.pdf

Zimmerman, M., Galione, J. N., Chelminski, I., Young, D., Dalrymple, K., & Ruggero, C. J. (2010). Sustained unemployment in psychiatric outpatients with bipolar disorder: Frequency and association with demographic variables and comorbid disorders. *Bipolar Disorders* 12:720–726.

8.3 CASE S: DISCHARGE OF A NEPHEW

8.3.1 Case

Mr. S. was a handsome young man who was admitted to a state hospital from a community hospital emergency room (ER).

Interview

On admission, Mr. S. claimed he was doing what was expected of him in the state clinic he attended, that is, he took his medication—divalproex and olanzapine—did not use illicit drugs, allowed bloodwork, and attended programs. His medications and his programs were okay. The problem he had was with his psychiatrist, Dr. B., who, he complained, was playing games and joking too much.

Mr. S. recalled spending time in a children's psychiatric hospital when he was still in grade school but couldn't say why. "I was just put there," he said, "they didn't tell me why. Every time I turned around I got put places. Everywhere I went, they were laughing at me." For years, on and off, he took divalproex but couldn't say why, just that he took it. He said that olanzapine helped him in his mind when his mind was telling him to do something stupid.

History

Dr. B. related that, earlier on the day that Mr. S. sought admission at the hospital ER, he had a scheduled appointment in the clinic. He said Mr. S. refused to allow bloodwork to measure his valproate level and that he was belligerent. Dr. B. said, "He threatened to kill me! He's assaultive! He's a substance abuser! He has poor impulse control!"

The medical records department retrieved old records from various children's hospitals. They were faintly yellow, covered with notes written with the broad strokes of a fountain pen or with the nubby indentations of a mechanical typewriter. Records documented a history of behavior problems starting at age 5. By age 11, Mr. S. had been admitted to a day hospital for aggressive outbursts at school, hyperactivity, inability to concentrate, and refusing to do any schoolwork. They noted that he stole from home, stayed out late at night, and set fires. His parents died when he was a toddler, so Mr. B. was raised by his grandmother. Staff reported that she minimized the boy's problems or blamed others. After the boy was suspended from a day hospital because he hit other children, his grandmother signed him out against medical advice (AMA). He was discharged on medication for attention deficit disorder.

Other records showed he had been arrested at least once almost every year since he was 17. Arrests were for a variety of crimes, but many were for assault.

Outpatient records began about a year before his current admission. Dr. B. first wrote that his patient admitted to marijuana and cocaine-crack abuse, which caused a continuing risk of violence, but he followed this note with one stating that Mr. S. understood if he did not present himself regularly to clinic his case would be terminated. Within a month of starting treatment at the clinic, Mr. S. was arrested for assault. Dr. B. prescribed olanzapine but stopped divalproex due to noncompliance with monitoring for therapeutic levels.

Three weeks after his divalproex was stopped, Mr. S. took himself to a community hospital ER asking to be admitted because he kept getting into fights. Psychiatrists noted auditory hallucinations telling him to hurt and kill others and beliefs that random people on the street talked about him. They also noted that Mr. S. slept 3–4 hours per night, then woke to pace and clean his room. And he had, by his admission, assaulted someone on the street the previous day. His urine toxicology screen was positive for cocaine and THC (marijuana), while his divalproex level was nearly nondetectable. ER psychiatrists transferred him to a state hospital.

Course of treatment

Mr. S. was restarted on divalproex in addition to olanzapine. He was asked to sit and listen in therapeutic groups, but he could not. Instead, he complained he was caged in, got angry and loud, and walked out. Every day, several times a day, he sought out his psychiatrist. He was complimentary and affectionate one minute, suspicious and angry the next. "When am I leaving?" he demanded, "I got things to do! You don't understand! I got court cases! You're playing with my mind!" The doctor asked him to give it a little more time. Mr. S. responded, "I'm gonna sue you! You're keeping me too long!"

Mr. S.'s grandmother had died years earlier, but he lived with his aunt. When his psychiatrist called her she reported that she had had no problems with her nephew; he never cursed or disrespected her. On the contrary, the young man went to church, cleaned his room, played video games, and in other ways kept busy about their home. She believed he was taking prescribed medication and not drinking or using street drugs. His doctor suggested he had some psychiatric problems; she replied, "We all do. There's plenty of young girls in the neighborhood don't think he's got a mental problem." His doctor asked about his criminal problems. "Water under the bridge," his aunt said, "People don't understand him."

Later, Mr. S.'s aunt appeared in the hospital to meet with his psychiatrist and team leader. She declared that he did not belong in the hospital, that changing his medication should not take more than 2 weeks. Besides, he didn't need psychiatry. What he needed was prayer and to be with his family. In the meeting, Mr. S. agreed. His aunt threatened to take Mr. S. home with her that day. But she did not, and Mr. S. did not ask to go with her. After she left, Mr. S. asked his doctor to please work with her.

As before, Mr. S. approached his psychiatrist at every sighting, anxious to be in court for his criminal cases and anxious about an application for Social Security benefits (SSI or Supplemental Security Income for disabled adults). He provided what information he could to help his social worker and doctor complete his application. He was still urged to attend groups. Restless, he drifted in and out of classrooms. He spent some time in a group for substance abusers, then a short time in a medication education group, where he cozied up to a female patient, then got up and walked out. He volunteered that he had trouble staying in groups because he had trouble concentrating, a life-long problem.

As his psychiatrist gradually increased his dose of divalproex, the constant pressing for discharge eased off; he felt calmer. The hallucinations had stopped, as did the belief that others laughed at him. Mr. S. knew he got into fights when he was not taking his medication; he said he needed to continue to take it and to stay away from illegal drugs.

He was discharged about 10 weeks after he was admitted with a court-ordered assisted outpatient treatment (AOT) plan that included residence with his aunt, treatment with divalproex and olanzapine, clinic follow-up with Dr. B., and an intensive case manager (ICM). His aunt was asked to consider joining a family support group at the clinic.

8.3.2 Comment

Mr. S. was lucky to have family who gave him affection and a home, showed up, and stood up for him. He was lucky to be able to work with both his treatment team and his aunt. He did not insist on leaving the hospital with her. By staying, he could take advantage of what it had to offer, which was, for him, psychiatric stability and a chance for a regular income (on SSI). With luck and continued stability, he could avoid jail and prison.

Mr. S. needed and accepted medication and an ongoing therapeutic relationship with Dr. B. His behavior problems seemed to be a consequence of bipolar disorder. If Dr. B. would work with him, if he would do his best to keep him in treatment and maintain his divalproex levels, he would do his part in controlling his illness and his behavior.

8.4 CASE T: DISCHARGE OF A BROTHER

8.4.1 Case

Mr. T. was a man in his 40s who was admitted to a state psychiatric hospital after being arrested on misdemeanor charges and found not fit to stand trial. His charges were dropped.

Interview

On admission, his psychiatrist met a disheveled man who could not say why he was sent to a hospital, though he did recall cursing and yelling at the judge at his court hearing. He endorsed trouble sleeping and occasional poor concentration for the previous several months, but his appetite and energy levels were fine; he was not hopeless and had not recently thought of suicide. However, he had experienced auditory hallucinations for the previous 6 years, through and including the day of admission. The voice of the devil told him to do bad things (e.g., hurt others and himself) and the voice of God told him to do good things (e.g., help others).

Substance abuse was also a problem in that he regularly drank too much alcohol and ingested heroin, cocaine, phencyclidine (PCP), and his prescribed methadone. Mr. T. admitted that he took his prescribed antipsychotic medication on an as-needed basis, to quiet the voices.

He said his first psychiatric hospitalization was in grade school because he was inattentive and rebellious in school and fought with other children. Later in childhood he was placed in a residential treatment facility. As an adult he was treated several times in prison and several times in a local community hospital for suicide attempts, depression, anxiety, manic-depression, and "cutting up" (deliberately cutting himself).

Both his parents were working people with stable jobs, but they could not provide their children a stable, safe, home life. After his father died due to a drug overdose, his mother took a common-law husband who frequently beat Mr. T. Mr. T. dropped out of high school but completed his GED and, later, in prison, college course work. His mother had died years earlier, but he remained close to a sister who had been sharing her home with him before he was arrested.

History

Fitness examiners noted that Mr. T.'s most recent arrest was one of many for misdemeanor nonviolent crimes. On their interview, he mumbled and rambled illogically about being King Tut and having been sent by God.

His outpatient bridger and his state clinic psychiatrist, Dr. C., also provided history. His bridger said he got up early in the morning to arrive at the apartment where Mr. T. lived in order to take him to clinic, but often not early enough. Mr. T. would frequently elude him. Dr. C. said that Mr. T.'s clinic chart had been closed because he quit showing up. When he did appear, he would refuse urine toxicology (illicit drug) screens and anything more than the most minimal communication with his psychiatrist. Dr. C. said that Mr. T.'s sister told him that her brother would not consistently bathe or eat meals but often walked around the apartment they shared intoxicated with multiple substances and confused. Nevertheless, Dr. C. said the sister did not seem alarmed and that he did not believe Mr. T. was a candidate for involuntary hospitalization.

Course of treatment

Mr. T.'s sister sat at a table in the conference room on the ward with Mr. T. and his treatment team. She was willing to have her brother live with her after discharge. "That's my brother; I love him," she said. But, she needed some support in caring for him, someone she could call for help. She was concerned about his illegal drug use and idleness. "He was a good guy who got caught up in drugs and got hold of the dust (PCP)," she said. She wanted him to get into psychotherapy so he could clear up issues inside himself and stay sober.

Mr. T. sat beside his sister, listened, and agreed. "Drugs were a big part of my life," he admitted. "I was gullible to them. I need a program for drugs and group therapy and individual therapy." He added, "You gotta start with being honest with yourself. I'm ready to try something new."

At the end of this meeting, the team had a plan to present to Mr. T. and his sister. It was a ambitious package including assisted outpatient treatment (AOT), which itself required an intensive case manager (ICM), long-acting injectable medication, a vocational program, a substance abuse program, and individual and group therapy, if available.

Later, when a resident in psychiatry and the ward attending asked more questions, Mr. T. revealed more. He said he was repeatedly and over the course of years sexually abused by a male family member. The abuse started when he was in grade school, a year or so before the voices started. While he was still disturbed by memories of childhood abuse, he was also troubled by other traumas he had suffered in his 20s, such as being attacked in prison and being shot on the streets.

Mr. T. experienced psychotic, mood, and posttraumatic stress disorder (PTSD) symptoms. He reported daily hallucinations that told him to cut himself, or that he was a king, or that his family member shouldn't have done that to him. He believed he was a king. In addition, he said he experienced pain and anguish and thought of cutting as a way of taking it out on himself. And he admitted to nightmares and to reexperiencing events.

Given this new information, his attending psychiatrist offered changes to his medication regimen. But, at this point, Mr. T. refused a long-acting injectable antipsychotic, explaining that it made him like a zombie. As his time on the ward passed, he grew impatient; he longed to return to the streets to take care of business and demanded discharge.

Plans for AOT; a case manager; and individual, group, and vocational therapy never materialized. Mr. T. wanted out, to live his life as he had before, and his sister did not object. So he was discharged back to his sister and to the outpatient clinic. On the day of discharge, he said the voices had been gone for about a week. They would come and go, but were not strong and didn't tell him so much negative things. His ideas about hurting himself were gone, so was his belief that he was a king.

8.4.2 Prevalence of reports of childhood abuse

A history of self-reported childhood maltreatment has been found to be highly prevalent among adults with serious mental illness who are treated in the US public psychiatry sector. Of a group of 569 adults with schizophrenia or schizoaffective illness treated in public systems, 56% reported childhood physical abuse, and 34% reported childhood sexual abuse (Rosenberg et al., 2007). Of 78 women who were being treated in a state operated clinic, 65% reported one of physical abuse, sexual abuse, or neglect (Munzenmazier et al., 1993). Fifty-eight percent were diagnosed with schizophrenia or schizoaffective illness.

8.4.3 Underrecognition of trauma

Tucker (2002) wrote that public-sector psychiatrists must not only detect and record a history of trauma but also consider that symptoms may have a traumatic etiology, as in PTSD. Flashbacks may be mistaken for hallucinations, shame may be seen as a delusion or guilt. (How childhood abuse may relate to auditory hallucinations is discussed in Chapter 3.6.) Patients with atypical presentations may be diagnosed with schizoaffective illness or psychosis not otherwise specified. Failure to recognize trauma and its possible sequela can result in poor treatment response and excessively long hospital stays.

8.4.4 What is a bridger?

Mr. T. had a "bridger," a state employee who provided a bridge between inpatient and outpatient services. A bridger establishes a relationship with a patient before discharge and then follows the patient after discharge to maximize the chances of a successful transition.

Bridgers are similar to workers who provide critical time intervention (CTI). To examine the outcome of CTI, a group of 150 discharged state hospital patients with a diagnosis of psychotic disorder and a recent history of homelessness were recruited from a state-operated transitional residence (Herman et al., 2011).

Those who agreed to participate were randomly assigned to usual care or to usual care with CTI after discharge from the transitional residence. CTI patients were offered 9 months of case management services focused on making the transition to community living. After 18 months, the CTI group had 1,812 homeless nights compared to 2,403 in the usual care group, a significant difference.

REFERENCES

Herman, D. B., Conover, S., Gorroochurn, P., Hinterland, K., Hoepner, L., & Susser, E. S. (2011). Randomized trial of critical time intervention to prevent homelessness after hospital discharge. *Psychiatric Services* 62(7):713–719.

Muenzenmaier, K., Meyer, I., Struening, E., & Ferber, J. (1993). Childhood abuse and neglect among women outpatients with chronic mental illness. *Hospital and Community Psychiatry* 44(7):666–670.

Rosenberg, S. D., Lu, W., Mueser, K. T., Jankowski, M. K., & Cournos, F. (2007). Correlates of adverse childhood events among adults with schizophrenia spectrum disorders. *Psychiatric Services* 58(2):245–253.

Tucker, W. M. (2002). How to include the trauma history in the diagnosis and treatment of psychiatric inpatients. *Psychiatric Quarterly* 73(2):135–144.

8.5 CHILDHOOD ABUSE AND ADULT MENTAL ILLNESS

8.5.1 Introduction

The studies outlined below present data on the association of childhood maltreatment with several adult psychiatric problems including posttraumatic stress disorder (PTSD), mood and anxiety disorders, substance abuse, antisocial personality disorder, suicidality, and violent crime. The studies also demonstrate that the risk of developing mental illness in adulthood is related to type of trauma, with sexual abuse a more powerful predictor; risk is, however, also related to individual vulnerabilities, childhood family environment, and adversities that occur after the abuse.

An early review (Browne & Finkelhor, 1986) noted long-term psychological effects of childhood sexual abuse. These are feelings of isolation and stigma, poor self-esteem, difficulty in trusting others, a tendency toward revictimization, and sexual maladjustment. These difficulties are not part of this discussion.

8.5.2 Officially reported child maltreatment

In one year, 2023, 0.74% (or 7.4 per 1,000) of the US population younger than 18 were victims of officially reported and substantiated child abuse or neglect (Children's Bureau, 2023). In 2016, an estimated 11.7% of US children had ever experienced officially reported and confirmed neglect or abuse by age 18 (Yi et al., 2020).

An analysis of official records of maltreatment of 1,193 children ages 5–13 (Vachon et al., 2015) revealed that neglect was the most common type of maltreatment, followed by emotional abuse, physical abuse, and sexual abuse. Sixty percent of children suffered more than one type of maltreatment. Sexual abuse was almost always accompanied by another type of maltreatment. Forty percent of the children experienced one or two episodes of maltreatment, while 23% experienced from 6 to 20. The most severe maltreatment each child suffered was classed as mild in fewer than 5% of cases, although in all cases maltreatment was serious enough to be officially reported. In 27% of cases, the maltreatment was severe.

8.5.3 Official reports versus self-reports

Prospective studies start with officially reported and confirmed cases, locate the victims in adulthood, and assess for mental illness. Retrospective studies ask adults to recall if they were maltreated in childhood and, at about the same time, assess for mental illness.

Retrospective self-reports lack the certainty of official reports. They are prone to forgetting. Forgetting may be related to the chronicity of the abuse, the age of the child when abuse occurred, the child's relationship to the abuser, and if abuse involved violence or threats of violence (Fergusson et al., 2000). Retrospective reports are also prone to misremembering. How adults recall events can be influenced by what they were told when they were children, and by how, as adults, they assess past events (Susser & Widom, 2012).

Adults with a psychiatric illness may be more likely to report a traumatic past in their search for a cause of their illness, an example of recall bias (Susser & Widom, 2012). Or reports can be prone to denial, that is, choosing not to report abuse due to embarrassment, shame, or reluctance to reactivate painful memories (Tucker, 2002).

Officially documented cases are far fewer than self-reported cases and may not be representative of all cases. In a survey of 23,395 Canadian households, 32% of adults reported a history of childhood physical or sexual abuse or of witnessing parental violence, but only 7.6% of adults who recalled maltreatment reported contact with child protection agencies (Afifi et al., 2015).

A prospective study (Widom & Czaja, 2012) identified a group of children who were abused and/or neglected according to official records and matched them to a control group. After the children grew into adulthood, they were assessed once, then again 10 years later. Twenty-nine percent of adults with a documented history of sexual abuse denied it at both assessments, 49% recalled it at both assessments, and 22% were inconsistent. Eight percent of the group with documented physical abuse denied it happened at both assessments, and 20% were inconsistent. At one assessment, some members of the control group without a documented history of child abuse reported abuse.

8.5.4 A retrospective study

As part of a larger study collecting information at intervals over the lives of all children born in Christchurch, New Zealand, over a four-month period, Fergusson and colleagues (2008) asked about 1,000 young adults to recall physical abuse by parents or sexual abuse before age 16 by anyone. At about the same time, investigators assessed the group for several psychiatric disorders, not including PTSD. They utilized data collected when the young adults were children on measures of IQ, family socioeconomic background, family functioning, and paternal behavior. This was an effort to separate out the effects of individual vulnerabilities (i.e., childhood IQ and gender and early family environment). Childhood maltreatment has been found to frequently occur with intercorrelated family problems, including parental substance abuse, parental criminality, parental mental illness, and family violence (Green et al., 2010).

Reports of either physical or sexual abuse were significantly associated with increased rates of psychiatric illness in young adulthood, including major depressive and anxiety disorders, conduct disorder/antisocial personality disorder, alcohol and other substance dependence, and suicidal ideas and behavior. Reported abuse was also significantly associated with total overall number of disorders.

However, physical and sexual abuse were significantly correlated with family and individual characteristics. After controlling for these variables, the relationship between history of physical abuse and later psychiatric problems became nonsignificant except for depression. For history of sexual abuse involving attempted or completed penetration, all relationships remained significant. Individuals who reported this type of abuse had overall rates of mental disorder that were 2.4 times higher than those without a history of sexual abuse.

Investigators estimated that exposure to any sexual abuse could account for 13.1% of all mental disorders in the group, while exposure to physical abuse accounted for 5.1%. This is the *population attributable risk*, the amount by which the rate of mental disorders would be reduced if sexual or physical abuse were eliminated.

8.5.5 A twin study

A retrospective study (Danielsdottir et al., 2024) began with 25,252 individuals age 18–47 years in the Swedish Twin Registry. Twins completed online surveys of childhood adversities: emotional or physical neglect; emotional, physical, or sexual abuse; rape, hate crime victimization; and witnessing family violence. Investigators then searched for members of the group in a nationwide database of records of inpatient and outpatient psychiatric treatment. Treatment after age 19 for depressive disorders, anxiety disorders, substance use disorders, and stress-related disorders was noted.

The risk of treatment for any of the above psychiatric illness was determined for those with exposure to childhood adversities compared to those without for the entire group. It was also determined for monozygotic and dizygotic twin pairs who were discordant for exposure to adversity (i.e., one was exposed to one or more adversities and the second was not). This method parses out the effect of shared family environment and of shared genes from the effect of trauma.

For the entire group, exposure to three or more adversities was associated with greater odds of treatment for any psychiatric disorder, with an odds ratio 4.57. For discordant dizygotic twins, the odds ratio was 2.25; for monozygotic twins, it was 2.11. For rape, the odds ratio was 3.68 for the full group, 2.48 for discordant dizygotic twin pairs, and 1.75 for discordant monozygotic pairs. These results indicate that an effect of three or more adversities or rape on later psychiatric disorder remained after controlling for shared genes and environment. In contrast, for physical abuse, the odds ratio for the entire group was 2.67, but 1.20 for discordant dizygotic twin pairs and 1.12 for discordant monozygotic pairs, indicating a minimal effect of the abuse.

8.5.6 A prospective study

In a prospective study (Widom, 1999), 908 children who had experienced court-substantiated physical or sexual abuse or neglect before age 12 were matched to 667 controls on the basis of age, race, and approximate socioeconomic status. Seventy-six percent of the original entire group of children were interviewed at mean age 29 to determine rates of various psychiatric disorders. Investigators also determined lifetime rates of other traumatic events, of other childhood family problems, and of other lifetime adversities.

Twenty-one percent of control participants met criteria for a lifetime PTSD diagnosis, while 31% of the abused and neglected group did—a significant difference. The odds ratio for lifetime PTSD for adults who experienced neglect compared to the control group was 1.72, for physical abuse 1.90, and for sexual abuse 2.34.

The maltreated group had significantly more childhood adversities, more lifetime adversities and problems, and more traumatic lifetime events overall than the comparison group. In an analysis including these variables, significant predictors of a lifetime PTSD diagnosis were behavior problems before age 15, having an alcohol or other substance abuse disorder diagnosis, and being separated, divorced, or widowed, but not childhood maltreatment.

The number of lifetime PTSD symptoms was related to childhood abuse or neglect and having a parent who was arrested or had a substance abuse problem, in addition to the same variables associated with PTSD diagnosis. A history of sexual abuse was a much more significant predictor of lifetime PTSD symptoms than was a history of physical abuse. Neglect was not a significant predictor.

Another analysis (Horwitz et al., 2001) considered the effect of childhood maltreatment on adult mental illness after controlling for lifetime stressors. Some stressors were job instability, unemployment, homelessness, and parental or sibling drug abuse or arrest. No difference was found in rates of dysthymia diagnosis for control women versus maltreated women. In men, childhood victimization was related to lifetime dysthymia diagnosis. The relationship remained even after controls for lifetime stressors.

Rates of diagnoses of lifetime alcohol abuse or dependence in men and women were not significantly different between maltreated and control groups. Lifetime stressors were strongly related to measures of alcohol abuse for men and women.

Rates of antisocial personality disorder (ASPD) diagnosis in both genders was more likely in the victimized group. In men, 27% of maltreated group had an ASPD diagnosis while 17% of control group did. However, the relationship between ASPD diagnosis and childhood maltreatment did not remain after controlling for lifetime stressors. Lifetime stressors were strongly related to ASPD diagnosis for both sexes.

These results may be related to socioeconomic status. Both maltreated and control groups were composed of people who grew up in poverty. Men living in poverty have high rates of alcohol abuse, while women have high rates of dysthymia.

An analysis of rates of arrest for violent crime (Widom & Czaja, 2012) considered the effect of different lifetime adversities and disorders, including a history of conduct disorder, marital instability, and a substance abuse diagnosis. Data from official arrest records dating from when subjects' average age was 33 showed that 21% of the group who had been mistreated had been arrested for a violent crime, compared to 16% of the control group (odds ratio of 1.44). However, the impact of child abuse and neglect became insignificant when controlling for other lifetime adversities and disorders. This suggests that being mistreated as a child is a marker for these other risk factors, or that being violent as an adult is not a direct result of childhood maltreatment but a result of the relationship between childhood mistreatment, conduct disorder, and substance abuse.

Another study (DuMont et al., 2007) concluded that many abused and neglected children grew up to be resilient as young adults. *Resilience* was defined as at least six of the following: high school graduation, being socially active, no psychiatric or substance abuse diagnosis, no arrests or self-reported violence, no employment problems, and no homelessness. Of the maltreated group, 30% met this criteria compared to 46% of the comparison group, a significant difference.

REFERENCES

Afifi, T. O., MacMilllan, H. L., Taillieu, T., Cheung K., Turner S., Tonmyr L., & Hovdestad W. (2015). Relationship between child abuse exposure and reported contact with child protection organizations: Results from, the Canadian Community Health Survey. *Child Abuse and Neglect* 46:198–206.

Browne, A., & Finkelhor, D. (1986). Impact of child sexual abuse: A review of the research. *Psychological Bulletin* 99(1):66–77.

Children's Bureau. (2023). An office of the Administration for Children & Families, U. S. Department of Health & Human Services. Child Maltreatment 2023. Accessed on October 12, 2025, from https://acf.gov/cb/data-research/child-maltreatment

Danielsdottir, H. B., Aspelund, T., Shen, Q., Halldorsdottir, T., Jakobsdottir, J., Song, H., . . . & Valdimarsdottir, U. A. (2024). Adverse childhood experiences and adult mental health outcomes. *JAMA Psychiatry* 81(6):586–594.

DuMont, K. A., Widom, C. S., & Czaja, S. J. (2007). Predictors of resilience in abused and neglected children grown-up: The role of individual and neighborhood characteristics. *Child Abuse and Neglect* 31:255–274.

Fergusson, D. M., Boden, J. M., & Horwood, L. J. (2008). Exposure to childhood sexual and physical abuse and adjustment in early adulthood. *Child Abuse and Neglect* 32:607–619.

Fergusson, D. M., Horwood, L. J., & Woodward, L. J. (2000). The stability of child abuse reports: A longitudinal study of the reporting behavior of young adults. *Psychological Medicine* 30:529–544.

Green, J. G., McLaughlin, K. A., Berglund, P. A., Gruber, M. J., Sampson, N. A., Zaslavsky, A. M., & Kessler, R. C. (2010). Childhood adversities and adult psychiatric disorders in the national comorbidity survey replication I: Associations with first onset of DSM-IV disorders. *Archives of General Psychiatry* 67(2):113–132.

Horwitz, A. V., Widom, C. S., McLaughlin, J., & White, H. R. (2001). The impact of childhood abuse and neglect on adult mental health: A prospective study. *Journal of Health and Social Behavior* 42:184–201.

Susser, E., & Widom, C. S. (2012). Still searching for lost truths about the bitter sorrows of childhood. *Schizophrenia Bulletin* 38(4):672–675.

Tucker, W. M. (2002). How to include the trauma history in the diagnosis and treatment of psychiatric inpatients. *Psychiatric Quarterly* 73(2):135–144.

Vachon, D. D., Krueger, R. F., Rogosch, F. A., & Cicchetti, D. (2015). Assessment of the harmful psychiatric and behavioral effects of different forms of child mistreatment. *JAMA Psychiatry* 72(11):1135–1142.

Widom, C. S. (1999). Posttraumatic stress disorder in abused and neglected children grown up. *American Journal of Psychiatry* 156(8):1223–1229.

Widom, C. S., & Czaja, S. J. (2012). Childhood trauma, psychopathology and violence: disentangling causes, consequences, and correlates. In *Trauma, Psychopathology, and Violence: Causes, Consequences, or Correlates?* Eds. C. S. Widom, pp. 291–317. New York: Oxford University Press.

Yi, Y., Edwards F. R., & Wildeman C. (2020). Cumulative prevalence of confirmed maltreatment and foster care placement for US children by race/ethnicity, 2011–2016. *American Journal of Public Health* 110(5):704–709.

9

DISCHARGE TO SUPPORTIVE HOUSING

Supportive housing serves discharged patients who cannot live with family. This chapter describes types of housing as well as programs and services that accompany housing. One case shows how unstable housing contributes to psychiatric instability. In another case, a man found a home and support services and lived a peaceful, satisfied life. In two other cases, the men can achieve neither housing nor psychiatric stability.

9.1 CASE U: YOU GOT TO BE ALERT ON THE STREETS

9.1.1 Case

Mr. U. was a man in his 30s who was arrested for a misdemeanor crime, found not fit to stand trial, and transferred to a state hospital.

Interview

On initial interview, Mr. U. was silly one minute, testy and dismissive the next. When asked what he thought "Don't cry over spilt milk" meant, he replied, "You tell me. What I think about ain't no spilt milk." In anticipation of mingling with other patients on a ward he said, "I hope nobody will cause trouble with me, because when they push me, there's nothing I can do, but do what I do."

He said that in the 8 months before his most recent arrest he had been released from a community hospital, then arrested and admitted to another community hospital. He was discharged, then lived for a few months in a rented room and attended a clinic where he received injections of medication. When he had enough of side effects such as pain in his buttocks and stiffness, he quit the shots and left for a trip to another state. Soon after his return he was arrested for a minor property crime and then hospitalized. After discharge he took medication for a few days, lost his home, stopped taking medication, and was arrested again.

He admitted to a distant history of smoking marijuana and a recent history of drinking beer every day when he had a chance. Beer helped him fall asleep.

History

Fitness examiners found a dirty, smelly, unkempt man who was mostly uncooperative, at times mute, and at other times laughing uproariously.

Mr. U.'s mother appeared at the hospital to see her son and provide history. From his high school years, his life was a series of hospitalizations and rehospitalizations, often preceded by arrests. He would often become ill after stopping oral medication. She knew it was happening again when he was out on the street laughing, walking, and grinning, in a silly mood, and talking to himself. At such times he told her he heard voices. She recalled that her son was often given intramuscular medication because he got tired of pills. He could say he had a problem with anger, but did not believe he needed psychotropic medication and complained of side effects such as dry mouth.

His mother also reported that Mr. U. was frequently admitted to a local community hospital and, as an outpatient, was followed by their assertive community treatment (ACT) team. The community hospital did not arrange for supervised housing but consistently discharged Mr. U. to his mother or sister. His mother would feed him and let him use her shower but did not allow him to stay with her because her current partner, not Mr. U.'s father, was opposed.

Course of treatment

Mr. U. often laughed as he paced the hallways and dayroom of the ward, but even as he laughed, he was angry. He had only disdain for his fellow patients and for clinicians who insisted he needed to stay and get treatment. The problem was other people and their annoying behavior, he told his psychiatrist, not his irritability. He clamored for discharge. He did not accept his doctor's suggestion that he was manic, had mood swings, or a temper problem, or that he needed a mood stabilizer. He said he could handle the outside world himself.

Despite his lack of insight he accepted divalproex and fluphenazine decanoate as prescribed. Bit by bit, over the course of 6 weeks and with persistence and cajoling, Mr. U. responded. He appeared on the ward in fresh white sneakers and crisp jeans. He stopped his restless pacing and became contained and focused, with a direct gaze and a lift in his step.

One day, Mr. U. sat with his doctor and described his day-to-day life outside of hospitals and jail.

He said he had a regular income from Social Security, which he would supplement by doing odd jobs for a small neighborhood business. He tried to live on his own in studio apartments, but couldn't because his money didn't add up to enough. He was often told, "Your sister's got an extra room. Move in with her." But his sister didn't want him there, and he didn't want to be there. They got into too many arguments. He would rent rooms from strangers. Some charged a lot, and they still wanted more money. It all came down to money, but he didn't have it.

So he slept on the streets. Once, in a park, his eyes were closed but a voice told him somebody's there. Somebody was leaning over him, looking at his bag. He took his bag. In there, he had his cans of food, his can opener, his deodorant, his clothes, his towels. If it weren't for that voice, he didn't know what could have happened. The man would have hit him if he woke up.

He said, "You got to be alert on the streets. Walking by a group on the street, you never know. An argument might break out. They might have a knife, a gun. You might get pulled into it. I can't be taking medication on the streets when I'm homeless. If it's too much, I won't be able to protect myself. It makes everything react slow. I can't react like I should. It makes me tired. I have to be living in a quiet, safe place to be taking medication."

Because Mr. U. could not live with his family, he was homeless. He was discharged to a supervised residence where he would have a quiet, safe place in which to take his medication. In addition, he was discharged with an outpatient commitment order and an intensive case manager.

9.2 HOUSING FOR SERIOUSLY MENTALLY ILL ADULTS

9.2.1 The process of placement

Mr. U. was placed in community housing, the end result of a process he and his social worker undertook of applications, tours, and interviews. He would have to agree to participate in a particular housing program and that program would have to agree to accept him. Programs screen to find applicants whose needs fit within the scope of their mission and their resources. Placement can be more difficult for state hospital patients who are medically ill or at risk for substance abuse (Silver & McKinnon, 1994) or violence. The sequence of applications and interviews can be repeated multiple times after multiple rejections, thus requiring several weeks—far longer than the average length of stay in most community hospitals.

Mr. U.'s social worker was motivated to find a good fit because the worker knew that if Mr. U. became dissatisfied with his new home, he would be free to walk away. And Mr. U., like most inpatients, was motivated to get out of the hospital and live as independently as possible.

9.2.2 Housing and housing programs

Community housing for seriously mentally ill adults can be characterized in several ways. It can be permanent or nonpermanent. Nonpermanent housing can be transitional, that is, a transition to permanent housing. Or it can be on a continuum, with tenants moving from more- to less-supervised settings as they show progress in recovery. Housing can be in units scattered across a community (*scatter-site*) or in a single building.

Housing programs are also variable. They offer a range of services in addition to housing, as part of a package, from meal plans, to treatment, recreation, and rehabilitation services. Tenants can meet with service providers where they live or at a separate site, or service providers can travel to tenants. Housing programs can be low- or high-demand for tenants; that is, they can condition acceptance or continued tenancy on desirable behaviors such as treatment participation or sobriety.

9.2.3 Assertive community treatment

Assertive community treatment (ACT) is a service that programs may bundle with housing. It is offered by clinicians who meet patients where they live. It was first described in 1980, as an alternative to state hospitals for adults with chronically disabling psychiatric illness (Stein & Test, 1980). In that early version, team members provided whatever assistance and teaching patients needed in community living and employment. They were available 7 days per week, 24 hours per day. Treatment was assertive in that team members traveled to the homes of patients when they did not appear at their jobs. In a randomized trial of this intervention, 130 patients who sought admission to a hospital operated by the state of Wisconsin were assigned to ACT or to treatment as usual, which was most often hospitalization and eventual discharge. The patients were followed for 12 months. Of the 58 patients assigned to treatment as usual and hospitalized, 34 (58%) were readmitted within 12 months. In the same 12 months, 6% of ACT patients were hospitalized.

Later, Bond and Drake (2015) identified the critical components of the current ACT model as in vivo service, assertive outreach, continuous coverage, direct and integrated service (i.e., not service by referral to other agencies), a holistic approach to patient needs (including medication management, housing, and finances), a multidisciplinary team that meets frequently, and a low patient–staff ratio (about 10:1).

9.2.4 Housing First and other housing programs

Housing First or Pathways to Housing is an established expression of the permanent supportive housing model, a model with defined key elements (Rog et al., 2014). Housing First holds that housing is a basic right; it comes first, before and without sobriety or program attendance. A key element of the model is that housing is not contingent on service participation; it is low-demand. Tenants are offered services based on their needs and preferences. Another element is integration. Mentally ill individuals are not segregated from the general population in separate buildings but live in scatter-site units. Another requirement of the model is that mentally ill tenants adhere to house rules that are no different from rules that bind tenants who are not mentally ill. And another element is affordability. Tenants pay no more than 30% of their income on rent.

Supported housing programs may not adhere entirely to key elements of the model. Siegel and colleagues (2006) described two programs. In both, tenants paid 30% of their income for rent. Tenants controlled 70% of their income but were expected to pay for utilities and food. In one, tenants lived in scatter-site apartments, usually alone. An ACT team met with tenants weekly to provide medication and money management, support, and treatment services. An ACT team was also available to residents 24 hours per day as needed. Recreational programs were offered at a central site. Staying sober and in treatment were not preconditions for housing. In a second program, tenants lived in one building where only 30% of units were set aside for seriously mentally ill adults. Available on-site voluntary services included case management and job training. Crisis services coordinating with a psychiatric emergency service were always available. Being clean and sober for 6 months was a precondition for housing.

Other housing programs offer single-site, congregate living. Some offer only basic custodial care and require tenants to access treatment and rehabilitative services at a clinic or elsewhere. These are called *board and care homes*, *group homes for adults*, or *boarding homes*. Twenty-six board and care homes in California described by Mares and colleagues (2002) provided housing and meals. Most also provided basic supervision, dispensing of medication, and laundry services but only limited transportation and personal care. The average age of the 154 residents in these homes was 58.4.

Supervised or community residences offer more services on-site and make more demands. Of nine such residences described by Siegel and others (2006), six were reserved for people with serious mental illness but without co-occurring substance abuse. Tenants had single or shared rooms or studio apartments in a building with common areas for eating, meeting, and recreational activities. They were given a regular allotment of cash for personal needs after they turned over their monthly income (usually Social Security) to program managers in exchange for meals and services. Each had a case manager and was strongly encouraged to attend an off-site day or rehabilitation program. Housing staff were available 24 hours per day. Loss of sobriety, which was closely monitored, resulted in mandatory substance abuse treatment or expulsion.

9.2.5 Outcomes with housing versus treatment as usual

Tenants can leave and never return, but outcome studies have consistently found that, compared to treatment as usual, supportive housing increases stability and decreases homelessness. A review of 14 studies (Benston, 2015) concluded that a majority of homeless mentally ill people who were placed in housing programs with case management remained in housing at least 1 year or were housed more days than they were unhoused compared to a comparison group.

A group in California (Gilmer et al., 2010) compared outcomes for 209 homeless seriously mentally ill adults placed in permanent housing with at least monthly meetings with ACT teams to outcomes for a matched control group of

154 provided only outpatient services. For the group in permanent housing, the mean number of days per year of homelessness declined from 192 during the year before placement to 62 in the year after placement. Comparing the year before and the year after initiation of the study showed that permanent housing with an ACT team significantly reduced use of services and criminal justice contact, by 14% for inpatient services, 32% for emergency services, and 17% for justice system contact. Housed individuals reported significantly better quality of life than the control unhoused group. For patients not placed in housing, use of emergency room services significantly increased, while hospitalizations and contact with police did not significantly change.

REFERENCES

Benston, E. A. (2015). Housing programs for homeless individuals with mental illness: Effects on housing and mental health outcomes. *Psychiatric Services* 66(8):806–816.

Bond, G. R., & Drake, R. E. (2015). The critical ingredients of assertive community treatment. *World Psychiatry* 14(2):240–242.

Gilmer, T. P., Stefancic, A., Etner, S. L., Manning, W. G., & Tsemberis, S. (2010). Effect of full-service partnerships on homelessness, use and costs of mental health services, and quality of life among adults with serious mental illness. *Archives of General Psychiatry* 67(6):645–652.

Mares, A. S., Young, A. S., Mc Guire, J. F., & Rosenheck, R. A. (2002). Residential environment and quality of life among seriously mentally ill residents of board and care homes. *Community Mental Health Journal* 38(6):447–458.

Rog, D. J., Marshall, T., Dougherty, R. H., George, P., Daniels, A. S., Ghose, S. S., & Delphin-Rittmon, M. E. (2014). Permanent supportive housing: Assessing the evidence. *Psychiatric Services* 65(3):287–294.

Siegel, C. E., Samuels, J., Tang, D.-,I., Berg, I., Jones, K., & Hopper, K. (2006). Tenant outcomes in supported housing and community residences in New York City. *Psychiatric Services* 57(7):982–991.

Silver, M. A., & McKinnon, K. (1994). Finding alternatives to the streets for the homeless mentally ill: Efficacy at a state hospital intensive placement unit. *Journal of Psycholinguistic Research* 23(1):67–73.

Stein, L. I., & Test, M. A. (1980). Alternative to mental hospital treatment. I. Conceptual model, treatment program, and clinical evaluation. *Archives of General Psychiatry* 37:392–397.

9.3 CASE V: WE'LL PICK HIM UP AND TAKE HIM HOME

9.3.1 Case

Mr. V. was a man in his 50s who was admitted to a state psychiatric hospital after his first and only arrest, for a misdemeanor assault. He was found not fit to stand trial, and his charges were dropped.

Interview

On admission, Mr. V.'s responses were relevant and coherent. His psychiatrist detected only minimal symptoms, which were a few strange beliefs, such that he could communicate with the dead, and occasional, not distracting, hallucinated voices calling his name. He believed he was arrested because he was mistaken for someone else.

At the time of his arrest he was regularly attending a clinic where he accepted a long-acting intramuscular antipsychotic drug, living in a supervised apartment program, and participating in Fountain House, a clubhouse where he had been a 15-year member. In his free time, he read about clairvoyance and religion and met with friends in his apartment to chat and drink coffee.

Before he found stable housing he had been living on the streets for years. Mr. V. said that during those years he was followed by large groups of thugs and members of an underground crime network, but this experience had not recurred since he was living indoors.

History

Fitness examiners noted inappropriate affect (i.e., a tendency to smile for no apparent reason) throughout his evaluation. His thinking was rambling and at times confused and illogical. Mr. V. said that he could predict winning lottery numbers. He admitted to occasional auditory hallucinations that were not commanding.

Old hospital records documented a history obtained at the time from the patient's father. Mr. V. Senior first noticed strange behavior in his son about 20 years before his current admission, when he lost his job and moved into his father's home from another state. When Mr. V. was not helping out in the small family business, he would crisscross his neighborhood passing out religious tracts of his own creation. His father did not share and did not understand Mr. V.'s religious beliefs. After a few years, Mr. V. Senior became seriously ill and sold his home and business. Having lost a family home, his son began living on the streets.

Records related that, after about 3 years on the streets, Mr. V. was brought by ambulance to an emergency room where medical staff found a malnourished, anemic, and unwashed man whose speech was so disorganized he could barely communicate. What medical staff could understand was delusional. From the community hospital where he was admitted and treated for psychiatric illness, he was transferred to a state hospital where, on admission, his speech was rambling and illogical. On the ward, he was frequently heard talking to himself. The state hospital discharged him to a supervised apartment program, a day program, and a clinic. For 15 years, he was not hospitalized again, until he was arrested and found not fit to stand trial.

Course of treatment

The day after he was admitted two employees from his supervised apartment program came to visit. They told his treatment team that in the 3 years they had known him he had never hurt anyone or himself or threatened to do so. He thinks he is a psychic, they said, and he talks and laughs to himself. But, unlike other residents, he never complained that staff or his neighbors stole from him. He cared for himself without a problem; he kept his apartment tidy, laundered his clothes, maintained his personal hygiene, managed his own funds, routinely attended Fountain House, and kept his appointments with his clinic psychiatrist. There was no recent change in his psychiatric condition. In fact, he was the same as always. They asked when he could be discharged. Friends at the residence were asking about him. "We'll come pick him up and take him home when he's ready," they said.

His clinic psychiatrist called Mr. V. an old friend. He reported that Mr. V. had been consistently attending clinic; that he was stable, at his baseline, with disorganized thinking only when he conversed at length; and that he believed in a delusional system with confused religious ideas. He was not paranoid. "When he gets out of the hospital, I want to see him again," the doctor said.

A manager at Fountain House said that Mr. V. had been participating daily for many years. She called him the nicest man, a passive man, a man who talked to himself at times but could make sense when approached. She and other program employees had been to court to press for his early release. They also visited him in jail, where they were disturbed to see him with a black eye. "Call me when he's ready for discharge," she asked. She volunteered to pick him up.

Within 2 weeks of admission Mr. V. was discharged back to his residence, to Fountain House and his outpatient clinic.

9.3.2 Comment

This case illustrates the best possible outcome for outpatient care in a clinic, a day program, and a supervised residence. Mr. V. found a home and a network of support, keys to his success in staying in treatment and in his residence.

Other individuals are not so lucky. In the following case, Mr. W. was rejected by his housing program because the agency made demands that he could not meet, such as sobriety. The happy-go-lucky guy, Mr. X., would often return to one adult home where he had a girlfriend, but once told inpatient staff that he found such residences depressing and at other times complained that he was threatened there by his neighbors. The state hospital where he was repeatedly admitted was safer. The hospital and its staff were comfortable and familiar. It was also where he turned up whether he wanted to or not after he stopped taking psychotropic medication.

9.3.3 Fountain House

Fountain House originated the clubhouse model of psychosocial rehabilitation. It started with a group of patients at Rockland State Hospital in New York who formed a mutual support and socialization group. A psychiatrist on staff, Hiram Johnson, encouraged the group because he understood patients' social isolation and need for friends. After they were discharged, many of the original group continued meeting and organized as We Are Not Alone (WANA), which first met in March 1944. The first president of the Board of Directors was a volunteer from

Rockland State Hospital, Elizabeth Schermerhorn. She was instrumental in purchasing a building for the group, called Fountain House. With the cooperation of the Director of Rockland State Hospital, Russell Blaisdell, the group met with state hospital patients and offered them help in finding lodging and jobs after discharge, along with an invitation to join WANA (Anderson, 1998).

WANA reorganized as Fountain House, which opened in 1948 as a social club. It was the sole such club until the National Institute for Mental Health (NIMH) funded the National Clubhouse Training Program in 1977. In 2018, there were 326 clubhouses in 33 countries (McKay et al., 2018).

Fountain House is a voluntary, therapeutic community in which participants, called "members," run the day-to-day operations of the organization. They make progress on meeting their personal goals through supported education, supported employment, social engagement, relationship building, and health and wellness programming. Fountain House supports members in finding housing and access to psychiatric and primary care (Fountain House, n.d.).

REFERENCES

Anderson, S. B. (1998). *We Are Not Alone: Fountain House and the Development of Clubhouse Culture*. New York: Fountain House Inc.

Fountain House. (n.d.). Our services. Accessed on October 13, 2025, from: https://www.fountainhouse.org/services

McKay, C., Nugent, K. L., Johnsen, M., Eaton, W. W., & Lidz, C. W. (2018). A systematic review of evidence for the clubhouse model of psychosocial rehabilitation. *Administration and Policy in Mental Health* 45:28–47.

9.4 CASE W: REJECTED BY HIS HOUSING PROGRAM

9.4.1 Case

Mr. W. was a man in his 40s who was admitted to a state hospital after his outpatient psychiatrist reported he had threatened to hurt people. Before he was hospitalized, he was living in a supervised apartment provided by Agency A.

Interview

On admission, Mr. W. was irritable and suspicious but coherent and cooperative. He couldn't say why he had landed in the hospital. He allowed that he had had some disagreements with his case manager in that he objected to attending program daily, but they settled on three times weekly. And he admitted that he had stopped taking his medication or just took it on and off. When asked why, he couldn't give a reason, but said he just felt like it at the time. He mentioned he could not speak openly to professionals about his personal life because it would harm him or because they wouldn't understand. No, he did not see a change in himself after he stopped medication, and no, he had never threatened anyone.

The psychiatrist did not detect delusions or hallucinations. Mr. W. said his mood was not so good because he could not see why he needed to be in the hospital. "My case manager thinks I need this rest, but I don't think I need to be here," he said. He promised to take his medication at all times. "I stopped for the hell of it," he said, with much regret. Still, he did not believe he had psychiatric problems. He could admit that he had committed crimes in the past but said he had changed.

History

Mr. W. had been arrested several times, mostly for nonviolent crimes, and had spent time in prison. One arrest occurred 5 years previously, after he was accused of threatening, but not hurting, another person. He was found not fit to stand trial and sent to a state hospital for restoration of fitness, but, due to disorganized thinking and paranoia, he could not be made fit and was "Jacksoned." After further treatment he was discharged to a community residence run by Agency A.

Course of treatment

Mr. W. acknowledged that he was not taking his medication before admission and that this led to readmission. He was less ready to admit that he drank to celebrate a major holiday and then stopped his medication and refused to leave his apartment, which was the report that the inpatient team social worker received from Agency A. The agency worker also confirmed that Mr. W. had earlier negotiated an agreement that he would attend his day program a few days per week, not daily.

Mr. W. was eager to return to his apartment and, after a few weeks in the hospital, seemed ready, but Agency A. had other ideas. They would take him into their residence but not into his supported apartment. Mr. W. argued that it was unfair, that the residence brought up small things he had done in the past to justify their decision, and that he could keep his apartment clean. He wasn't drinking he said, but, yes, he did stop his medication.

Later, after weeks of uncertainty and a change in management staff at the residence, Agency A. reversed its decision and declined to accept Mr. W. back into its program at any level. He interviewed with another agency which also refused him. Finally, Mr. W. took a bed in the hospital's on-grounds residence.

Before he left, he was interviewed to assess his risk in the community. When asked about the crime for which he was arrested 5 years earlier, he said he would not repeat such behavior because he had an income from Social Security (SSI) and a stable living situation. He also said it was a mistake to stop his antipsychotic medication.

9.4.2 Ten years later

Mr. W. was admitted to a different state hospital for fitness restoration after he was accused of a crime similar to the one for which he was arrested several years earlier involving a threat of violence.

History

After his discharge 10 years earlier he continued treatment at his outpatient clinic for about a month. Within 3 years, he was hospitalized in another state hospital. About 7 years later, he was found by a psychiatric outreach team living in an isolated spot under a major highway. For a while they met with him regularly, bringing food and water and trying to establish trust. When they noticed new weakness in his left arm and leg, they called an ambulance and he agreed to be taken to a local community hospital.

At the hospital neurologists diagnosed a right hemisphere infarct. After a course of physical therapy they transferred him to the care of psychiatrists who gave him long-acting injectable antipsychotic medication, petitioned for assertive community treatment (ACT) services, and discharged him to a transitional living residence. When he entered the residence he was polite but guarded, with little to say. After 6 months, he was arrested.

Course of treatment

Mr. W. looked much older than his age, a lot worse for the wear; he held his left arm flexed and mostly useless at his side. He had little affect, and his speech was slow and sparse. Nurses described him as a model patient who always took his medication and bothered nobody. He kept to himself, with nothing to say in groups and only a few requests to his social worker: "When will I leave here? What will happen with my case? Will you call my lawyer?"

9.5 CASE X: A HAPPY-GO-LUCKY GUY

9.5.1 Case: In middle age

Mr. X. was a middle-aged man who was admitted to a state hospital after he violated an order of protection.

Interview

On admission, his psychiatrist met a physically unimposing man who was calm, controlled, and happy—happy to be where he knew most of the staff and patients. While he voiced some unusual beliefs in ancient Greek gods and extraterrestrials, he was otherwise logical and coherent and denied hallucinations. When asked about his mental problems, Mr. X. said he was bipolar, which to him meant that he had highs and lows; he agreed that a mood stabilizer helped him but added that he was just always a happy-go-lucky guy.

Mr. X. explained that he went to visit his family, but because they had obtained a legal order of protection from him, they called police. As Mr. X. related, his brother became upset with him because he asked for money he thought he was due. No, he said, he did not get angry with his family and, no, he had never forgotten to take his medications in the previous few months.

Mr. X. said he wanted to be admitted because he feared for his life due to harassment from another man living with him in the state hospital's on-grounds residence. He said he had left to walk the streets alone at night, hopeless, helpless, and scared.

History

This hospitalization was one of many for Mr. X. The first occurred when he was in his mid-20s. After discharge, he rebounded to the extent that by his early 30s, he was a well-educated man living independently and attending an outpatient clinic. A few months after he stopped showing up at the clinic he was arrested, found not fit to stand trial, and admitted to a state hospital. On one of his family's regular visits, his mother said the family wanted to help Mr. X. recover from his illness.

His later 30s and 40s brought many more hospitalizations. In between hospital stays, Mr. X. resided on the streets or in adult homes but never in one home for more than a few years. One, where he had a girlfriend, was an exception, in that he would return there frequently after hospitalizations. As he confided to a hospital psychology intern, adult homes, with their geriatric population, were depressing. Hospitals were preferable.

He was admitted several times to the same state facility. Sometimes he returned after he visited his family and they called police, or after he was threatening and destructive at his adult home. The hospitalization that occurred before his current one was particularly prolonged. He was admitted after he was arrested for a misdemeanor crime and found not fit to stand trial. In the hospital, his mood rapidly shifted between irritable and elated; he would shout threats and racial slurs at those around him and curse at his family over the phone. With medication, he slowed down, but he skipped doses, then stopped and returned to rage and threats. His psychiatrist petitioned for and was granted treatment over objection. Consistent medication led to remission of his mania and discharge after an extended stay. Six months later, he was readmitted.

Course of treatment

Mr. X. was cheerful, but not elated and not irritable. Back in the hospital, he was like a fish in water. Friendly, charming, and well-liked by all, he was adept at enlisting sympathy and securing small loans for coffee and snacks.

He said he was scared because one of the tenants in the group home was a big man who was bullying others for cigarettes, especially on weekends when staffing was thin. But he recognized that he was admitted to hospital because his family complained about his behavior. "Some of them want to see me in the hospital forever," he said. "I have no one else. I've done a lot for them in the past."

A brother agreed to meet with Mr. X.'s treatment team, though not with Mr. X.; at the arranged time, the brother did not show up. Mr. X. felt disappointed and abandoned. Though he understood that he had to leave his family alone, he missed them.

After a relatively short stay, Mr. X. was discharged to an adult home with an assisted outpatient treatment (AOT) order.

9.5.2 Twenty years later

When Mr. X. was past age 65, he was admitted to another state hospital for fitness restoration after he was arrested for a property crime. At the time of his arrest, he was living in a residence on the grounds of the state hospital where he had been treated 20 years earlier, and he was followed by an assertive community treatment (ACT) team. Before he came to the state hospital, he was held in jail. Clinicians there noted that he seemed just about normal until he stopped taking medications. He then gradually became easily enraged, spat at people, flooded his cell by flushing clothing down his toilet, and smelled of urine.

History

After he was discharged 20 years earlier, he told his clinic psychiatrist he felt well and optimistic about his treatment and about an AOT order, which he agreed to, saying he needed structure because he had been out of control of his life. He was also satisfied with his medications. Although almost immediately he complained of adverse effects, he continued medication for several months. Then he turned up at a community hospital emergency room complaining of fear of his new roommate and reporting he had been off medication for 2 weeks. All symptoms quickly resolved after admission.

Several more hospitalizations ensued, one after he threatened a family member and one after he was beaten and robbed. His clinic psychiatrist wrote that, given his frequent noncompliance, he might benefit from long-term hospitalization.

Over the years, Mr. X. would frequently disappear from his adult home and turn up in one of a number of hospital ERs, some in distant states. He was often seen and released. On one of his long-distance motor trips, he was involved in an accident that left him seriously injured.

Course of treatment

Soon after he was admitted, Mr. X. turned away when asked questions and cursed and spit at employees on his ward. He first refused medication, but later took it, and, after a few weeks, could focus and answer questions. Ward attendants complained that he harassed them with frequent requests for coffee and told them that because he was elderly he should be treated as special. On the ward, he spent his time by himself reading local newspapers. He forbade his social worker to talk with his family.

After he had been accepting treatment for a number of weeks he was interviewed by his treatment team. He remembered the state hospital where he had been treated many years earlier and its on-grounds residence. "Can I go back?" he asked. Then, in his next sentence, he recalled how he had to take long trips in a crowded van to get to a day program. Pushing out his elbows he showed how cramped he was. Nevertheless, he repeated, "I want to go back." When his interview completed, he spoke to the group assembled: "Thank you. Have a nice weekend everybody." Mr. X. pulled himself up from his chair and slowly and laboriously limped out the door.

Mr. X. was found fit to stand trial and returned to jail and then to court to face his charges.

10

DISCHARGE PLANNING AND RISK ASSESSMENT

Discharge decisions are guided by an obligation to meet the patient's needs in the least restrictive setting. Discharge plans must also maximize the chances that the patient and others will be safe. To accomplish the latter, clinicians must decide who is at risk for dangerous behavior and what kind of supervision can mitigate that risk. The chapter includes a summary of the literature on risk factors for violence in adults with psychiatric illness. In two cases, patients had needs that were difficult to meet in the community. In a third, a man needed supervision due to his risk of hurting others.

10.1 CASE Y: ANXIOUS AS LONG AS HE COULD REMEMBER

10.1.1 Case

Mr. Y. was a man in his 40s who was transferred to a state psychiatric hospital from prison on the day he completed his entire sentence for a property crime.

Interview

On admission, Mr. Y. said he had only heard voices when using drugs and had never been suicidal. He was under a lot of stress in prison, particularly since learning he had a serious chronic medical illness; he was anxious, scared, and depressed. With pains and shocks going through his body due, he was sure, to his illness, he couldn't sleep. Prison psychiatrists tried, but all the medications they prescribed to ease his distress didn't do much of anything for him.

He said he had been anxious as long as he could remember. And, as long as he could remember, he had functioned marginally and only with assistance. He was placed in special education classes for slow learners, then dropped out of school as soon as he could. As a young adult, he began drawing Supplemental Security Income (SSI). Before his most recent arrest, he was living alone in a single-room occupancy (SRO) hotel and drawing income from a variety of sources including SSI, welfare, an off-the-books physical labor job with a relative's small business, and shoplifting. His parents and siblings were deceased.

His history of previous treatment outside of prison was minimal, with only one previous hospitalization related to opiate abuse. The longest he had ever stayed in substance abuse treatment was 2 weeks, though he had been using his drug of choice, heroin, since his teens. Before he was arrested he was injecting heroin daily, using cocaine on weekends, and drinking a few beers now and then.

History

The prison that had released him sent a clinical summary from a psychiatrist stating that Mr. Y. said he heard voices in prison and also when he used cocaine. The prison also sent a summary of his criminal history that documented many, many arrests, starting in his teens, most for misdemeanor property crimes.

Mr. Y. had been released on parole on his conditional release date but was reincarcerated because he failed to meet a condition of his parole, which was to complete a substance abuse treatment program. Therefore, he was held until his maximum expiration date, the date on which he completed his entire sentence.

Course of treatment

On the ward, Mr. Y. did not voice delusions, admit to hallucinations, or behave bizarrely. He did have unrelenting anxiety, mostly expressed in fears for his physical condition. He immediately started a daily pressure campaign for methadone, insisting he would revert to intravenous heroin without some small maintenance dose to keep him happy. The state hospital could continue methadone but was not licensed to start it, so Mr. Y.'s psychiatrist could not accede to pressure. Instead, the doctor prescribed other medications for depression and anxiety, amitriptyline and olanzapine. When the low dose of olanzapine was stopped out of concern for adverse effects, Mr. Y. wanted it resumed.

Within a few weeks, Mr. Y. was preoccupied with how and when he could be discharged. His preference was to live by himself, in an SRO hotel. He had no patience for drug treatment programs. He wanted methadone, but he did not qualify for a methadone program because he was not using any opiates at the time. He insisted that he could not walk away from his residence because he needed his medication to live. And so Mr. Y. was discharged to the hospital's on-grounds residence where he could wait for a bed in a SRO hotel.

Return

Within 2 weeks, Mr. Y. was readmitted after he reported that he was depressed and suicidal. On admission, he related that he finally got his methadone by buying "spit out" (i.e., another resident's surreptitiously spit-out methadone dose). On top of methadone, he snorted a little heroin and drank a few beers.

Within a day he said he was not suicidal but hopeless, down and out, and disappointed that he could not quickly get Medicaid and his own room. His anxiety returned with him. He approached his psychiatrist several times a day with more physical complaints. At times, he could say that his medical illness had changed his life, that he felt less independent because of the many pills he had to take for his health. With an increase in amitriptyline to 150 mg/day he gradually approached his psychiatrist less often and had fewer and less-pressured complaints. His new discharge plan was to a specialized residence for people with serious medical conditions, substance abuse problems, and mental illness. The on-grounds residence was not for him.

10.1.2 Comment

In keeping with the Olmstead decision, Mr. Y. could not be held against his will in the hospital if community supports were appropriate and available. Appropriate community supports had to meet his individual needs and recognize his strengths. Before he was destabilized by his medical diagnosis and incarceration, he was able to live by himself and care for himself with the assistance of Social Security and welfare. To get him restabilized and not dependent on a hospital or supervised congregate living, he needed help in living with his medical condition, limiting his anxiety, and curtailing or at least minimizing the harm of his substance abuse.

Mr. Y. was unhappy with his community placement and so found his way back to the state hospital. He was lucky that community supports appropriate for him were available—but they were not readily available. Specialized housing was in high demand, so his social worker had to complete applications and Mr. Y. had to wait.

10.1.3 Notes on the Olmstead Decision

Discharge decisions are guided by multiple obligations—to optimize treatment, maximize the chances that the patient and others will be safe, and meet the patient's needs in the least restrictive setting.

The Olmstead Decision is an application of the 1990 Americans with Disabilities Act (ADA), which guarantees the rights of disabled people to live and be treated in the least restrictive setting necessary. The decision found that a state hospital in Georgia violated the ADA by involuntarily confining two women with developmental disabilities and psychiatric illness. One was Lois Curtis (LC), a 27-year-old woman who had spent most of her life, from age 11, in state hospitals (Roberts, 2022). The *Olmstead v. LC* case (1999) upholds the right of people with disabilities to supports and services in the community rather than in institutions as long the person does not object to community living, the person's treating professionals determine that community supports are appropriate, and community services are a reasonable accommodation (Sloan & Gulrajani, 2019).

REFERENCES

Americans with Disabilities Act of 1990 (ADA). 104 Stat. 337,42 U.S.C. 12132 (1990).

Olmstead v. L.C., 527 U.S. 581 (1999).

Roberts, S. (2022). Lois Curtis, whose lawsuit secured disability rights, dies at 55. November 10. *New York Times*. Accessed on October 13, 2025, from: https://www.nytimes.com/2022/11/10/us/lois-curtis-dead.html

Sloan, L., & Gulrajani, C. (2019). Where we are on the twentieth anniversary of *Olmstead v.* L.C. *Journal of the American Academy of Psychiatry and the Law* 47:408–413.

10.2 CASE Z: A MAN WITH INSULIN-DEPENDENT DIABETES

10.2.1 Case

Mr. Z. was a man in his 40s with insulin-dependent diabetes who was admitted to a state hospital after he allegedly pushed a staff member at his adult home, Home B.

Interview

On admission, Mr. Z. was a neat, somewhat irritable man whose speech was coherent and logical. He did not show delusional thinking and denied hallucinations and suicidal thinking. He was in the hospital because they sent him here, he said. Before this happened he had been living in a "mentally ill place." When asked if he had a mental illness, he admitted, "A little bit."

History

Mr. Z. dropped out of high school and never held a job. As a teenager he was first hospitalized for paranoia and hallucinations at the same facility where he was currently admitted. Almost every year, he was readmitted to the same hospital until he was in his late 20s, when he was admitted and retained for several years. He was discharged to Home B. and remained there for several years, leaving only for a few short-term admissions to community hospitals.

Course of treatment

His treatment team social worker promptly contacted staff at Home B. and was told that Mr. Z. got into an argument and pushed a staff member, but that they were willing to consider taking him back. Home B. had provided a critical service for Mr. Z. by arranging for a visiting nurse to check his blood glucose level and administer insulin on site. He was not trusted to do either on his own.

Mr. Z. was generally cheerful, comfortable in the hospital, and familiar with many employees there. He offered no complaints, and no one complained about him. At times he laughed for little reason, seemingly in reaction to his own internal world. While some attendants reported he admitted to hallucinations, Mr. Z. said it wasn't so. Later he said it was so, but he heard voices only about weekly, voices that sometimes told him bad things about himself but never told him to hurt anyone. Psychiatrists and other staff who remembered him could discern no significant change in him from the time he was discharged years earlier.

His psychiatrist's job was to work with the team internist to maintain or improve his psychiatric condition while decreasing or even eliminating his insulin requirements. On admission he was on a long-acting injectable antipsychotic agent, on which he had been discharged years earlier, but also olanzapine. The psychiatrist switched to another oral agent less likely to cause hyperglycemia. With this change the internist was able to cut his insulin requirements but did not succeed in eliminating his need entirely. Mr. Z.'s psychiatric condition remained the same. At times he was silly, at other times irritable. In therapeutic groups, he attended but made no meaningful contribution; his mind seemed elsewhere.

After some time passed it was clear Home B. would not allow Mr. Z. to return. He was left waiting and the team social worker was left with the job of finding a place that would care for his nursing needs.

Mr. Z. was given privileges to move off his ward independently during certain hours. He was coached to return to his ward on time, stick to his diet, and not panhandle in front of the snack bar. He returned to his ward on time but became a regular customer at the snack bar and also at vending machines, and so required more insulin.

After an interview at a group home he was not accepted; nor was he accepted at another, similar home. Mr. Z's treatment team could not be certain why he was rejected but concluded that he clammed up, turned shy or anxious, and put off interviewers who wanted something more or something different. After weeks and more rejections, the search was still on. Undaunted, the social worker submitted applications to a wider range of adult homes.

10.2.2 Comment

This patient, like Mr. Y., the man who was anxious as long as he could remember, could not be held against his will in the hospital if community supports to meet his individual needs were appropriate and available, but they were not.

10.2.3 Notes on the prevalence of general medical problems

Compared to the general population several medical disorders are more prevalent in adults with schizophrenia and other serious psychiatric illnesses (Janssen et al., 2015). When patients cannot participate in their own medical care (e.g., attend outpatient clinics, take medications, or administer insulin), they have a compromised ability to care for themselves. If supportive services are available, they may live in the community. But if services are not available, or if patients do not meet service providers' acceptance criteria, they can remain in hospital care. In 2001, Fisher and colleagues wrote that state hospitals treat and care for people with a complicated mix of psychiatric, medical, behavioral, and neurologic problems (Fisher et al., 2001).

Chronic obstructive pulmonary disease (COPD), hepatitis B and C, and HIV are all more prevalent in adults with serious mental illness than in the overall US adult population. So are obesity, hyperlipidemia, and hypertension, risk factors for coronary heart disease (CHD) (Janssen et al., 2015). It follows that death due to CHD occurs more commonly in people with schizophrenia compared to the general population (Hennekens et al., 2005). Another risk factor is cigarette smoking. People with schizophrenia, major depressive disorder, and bipolar disorder are more likely to be cigarette smokers than the general population (Hu et al., 2025).

REFERENCES

Fisher, W. H., Barreira, P. J., Geller, J. L., White, A. W., Lincoln, A. K., & Sudders, M. (2001). Long-stay patients in state psychiatric hospitals at the end of the 20th century. *Psychiatric Services* 52(8):1051–1056.

Hennekens, C. H., Hennekens, A. R., Hollar, D., & Casey, D. E. (2005). Schizophrenia and increased risks of cardiovascular disease. *American Heart Journal* 150(6):1115–1121.

Hu, Z., Cui, E., Chen, B., & Zhang, M. (2025). Association between cigarette smoking and the risk of major psychiatric disorders: A systematic review and meta-analysis in depression, schizophrenia, and bipolar disorder. *Frontiers in Medicine (Lausanne)* 12:1529191. doi: 10.3389/fmed.2025.1529191. eCollection 2025

Janssen, E. M., McGinty, E. E., Azrin, S. T., Juliano-Bult, D., & Daumit, G. L. (2015). Review of the evidence: Prevalence of medical conditions in the United States population with serious mental illness. *General Hospital Psychiatry* 37(3):199–222.

10.3 CRITERIA FOR INVOLUNTARY COMMITMENT

From the nineteenth century onward, commitment criteria were simply that a person be mentally ill and in need of treatment. This changed in the 1960s and 1970s, when laws and courts started to recognize patients' right to liberty and to due process in commitment proceedings. In 1964, Congress changed commitment criteria for the District of Columbia to mentally ill and dangerous to self or others (Appelbaum, 1994). In 1969, California set initial commitment criteria as dangerous to self or others or gravely disabled (i.e., unable to provide for basic needs) as a result of mental illness. Criteria for an additional 90 days retention was "imminently dangerous" (Abramson, 1972).

In 1971, police officers in Wisconsin picked up Alberta Lessard from in front of her house and took her to a local mental health center where she was admitted involuntarily. Three days later, without Ms. Lessard present, the officers appeared before a judge to explain why she should be detained longer. She was detained for another 10 days. Later, a psychiatrist from the mental health center recommended permanent commitment, and again, without her presence, a judge ordered further retention. With representation from Milwaukee Legal Services, Ms. Lessard brought suit in federal court (Appelbaum, 1994).

The *Lessard v. Schmidt* ruling of 1972 determined that criteria for retention are mental illness and imminent dangerousness to self or others beyond a reasonable doubt. Dangerousness must be based at minimum upon a recent act, an attempt, or a threat to do substantial harm. Psychiatrists who testify for involuntary retentions must also demonstrate beyond a reasonable doubt that alternatives to hospitalization are unsuitable or unavailable.

In 1975, the Supreme Court made a similar ruling in *O'Connor v. Donaldson.* Kenneth Donaldson had been involuntarily confined in a Florida state hospital for almost 15 years. His doctor refused to release him to the care of a friend or to a halfway house employee (Kopolow, 1976). The Court ruled that a state cannot confine a person against his or her will who is not dangerous and who is capable of surviving safely in the community either independently or with the help of others.

By the end of the 1970s, all US states restricted involuntary commitment to people dangerous to themselves or others, including dangerousness as manifested by inability to care for basic needs. Though the American Psychiatric Association was initially supportive of restrictive commitment laws, by the early 1980s, it reversed its position (Appelbaum, 1994). Individual psychiatrists articulated opposition to restrictive criteria based on its effect on severely ill patients and on the practice of public psychiatry. In his letter, "Dying with Their Rights On," the superintendent of a Wisconsin state hospital (Treffert, 1973) cited cases of patients who died because they did not meet his state's narrow criteria for involuntary hospitalization. Peszke (1975) argued that limiting treatment to those who are sick and dangerous means those who were sick but not dangerous are abandoned because they cannot help themselves due to impaired rational and executive functioning. Abramson, a consultant to a California county jail system, wrote (1972) that mentally ill people were being arrested and prosecuted for minor crimes so they could be detained because police knew that they were unlikely to be held in psychiatric hospitals. Peszke (1975) also argued that prediction of dangerousness is not and should never be within medical competence because the psychiatrist's sole aim is to protect the patient, not society. He acknowledged that societal concerns are important but wrote that they should be dealt with by the judicial system.

Broader criteria can prevail. Evidence shows that narrow commitment criteria have been stretched to accommodate what clinicians, attorneys, judges, and family members believe are patients' best interests. In law, commitment criteria have been expanded in several states (Appelbaum, 1974). For example, as of 2025, in the state of Washington, involuntary treatment can be justified by risk of harm to people or property, or of a severe deterioration in routine functioning shown by increasing loss of control over behavior in a person not receiving care essential for their health and safety (Washington State Health Care Authority, 2024). In *Selzer v. Hogue* (1993), a judge ruled that a patient's past behavior can factor into retention decisions. Larry Hogue was a New York state citizen with a history of schizophrenia and polysubstance abuse and many involuntary psychiatric admissions and incarcerations for dangerous behavior. After he was committed to a hospital, his behavior improved and he petitioned for release. His psychiatrist testified that he was not suitable for any outpatient treatment program and that, if released, he would be nonadherent, his condition would deteriorate, and he would become dangerous, as had happened many times before. The judge ruled for involuntary retention.

REFERENCES

Abramson, M. F. (1972). The criminalization of mentally disordered behavior: Possible side-effect of a new mental health law. *Hospital and Community Psychiatry* 23(4):13–17.

Appelbaum, P. S. (1994). *Almost a Revolution: Mental Health Law and the Limits of Change*. New York: Oxford University Press.

Kopolow, L. E. (1976). A review of major implication of the *O'Connor v.* Donaldson decision. *American Journal of Psychiatry* 133(4):379–383.

Lessard v. Schmidt, on remand, 379 F. Supp. 1376 (E. D. Wis. 1974).

O'Connor v. Donaldson, 422 U. S. 563 (1975).

Peszke, M. A. (1975). Is dangerousness an issue for physicians in emergency commitment? *American Journal of Psychiatry* 132(8):825–828.

Seltzer v. Hogue, 187 A.D.2d 230, 594 N.Y. S.2d 781 (N.Y. App. Div. 1993).

Treffert, D. A. (1973). Dying with their rights on. *American Journal of Psychiatry* 130(9):1041.

Washington State Health Care Authority. (2025). Involuntary Treatment Act (ITA). Accessed October 16, 2025, from: https://www.hca.wa.gov/assets/program/fact-sheet-involuntary-treatment-act.pdf.

10.4 CASE AA: A MAN NEEDS SUPERVISION

10.4.1 Case

Mr. AA. was a man in his 50s who was admitted to a state hospital less than 2 weeks after he was discharged from that same hospital to live with his son. He was admitted after his intensive case manager (ICM), part of his assisted outpatient treatment (AOT) team, brought him into a state clinic for evaluation. There a psychiatrist found him with alcohol on his breath, malodorous, disheveled, irritable, and muttering threats.

Interview

At the state hospital his psychiatrist met a sad and sluggish man with downcast eyes. The doctor asked what went wrong with his discharge plan. Mr. AA. said he never could get in touch with his son, so he moved in with his uncle. When he attempted to withdraw money from his bank account, he discovered that his son had gotten there first and cleaned him out. He said his ICM was no help; she didn't move fast enough to help him find an apartment. Despite these setbacks, he was ready with a plan: find his ICM worker, learn what she wanted him to do, and live with a second son.

History

For the previous 25 years, Mr. AA. had had multiple psychiatric hospitalizations for treatment of symptoms of schizophrenia, including auditory hallucinations, disorganized thinking, and delusions, particularly paranoid delusions about dark-skinned people he believed were of Indian or Pakistani descent. The state hospitalization that ended with discharge to an ICM and AOT was triggered by an arrest for assault. The hospitalization immediately preceding ended with discharge to a residence for adults with substance abuse and other serious mental illness, along with an appointment to a clinic where he would get regular injections of long-acting antipsychotic. That discharge plan failed when he walked out of the residence and quit attending the clinic.

For the previous 25 years, Mr. AA. had been in and out of jail. He had been arrested many times for mostly nonviolent crimes but also for a few that were violent and serious. His substance abuse history began in his late teens, when he began using intravenous heroin and cocaine, marijuana, and alcohol. Though he had stopped using illicit drugs several years before his current admission, he was still drinking alcohol to excess.

Course of treatment

On a long-acting injectable antipsychotic, Mr. AA. soon returned to the level of functioning and symptoms he had reached before his previous discharge. When he learned that his uncle died suddenly, he was tearful but able to talk about his feelings and continued attending groups, keeping himself clean and well dressed, and communicating easily. One week he apologized for drinking after discharge, but the next week he made light of it, saying it was just beer.

And so began a drawn-out negotiation around discharge plans. Mr. AA. insisted he did not need to be in the hospital and that he had a place to stay, with his second son. The ward social worker and psychiatrist knew that this was the same man who had refused him a home at his last discharge and had substance abuse problems of his own. Team members individually and in a group told Mr. AA. that they would talk with any family member or friend who would appear to discuss his discharge, but pressed the idea of a supervised residence because he had stayed sober and non-psychotic in a supervised residence in the past.

He promised that his son would appear, but, on the appointed day, he did not. His next plan was to live with a friend. "Have him come meet with the team," his social worker proposed. "He is old and can't move around and can't travel," Mr. AA. replied. "He can't keep an eye on you," his worker told him. "I am an adult and do not need supervision," he said, "I am here for one little beer. Drinking is not a problem for me."

Finally, Mr. AA. relented. While he accepted a supervised residence, he still longed for closer relationships. He held on to the hope that he might marry a girlfriend after he, as he put it, "polished up their relationship."

But before he could be discharged he needed a risk assessment and clearance by a hospital committee. A risk assessment required a better understanding of his history of violence. His treatment team talked with him about the times in the previous 20 years he had been arrested for hurting people. He recalled hitting and hurting a man sitting next to him in a bar who looked Indian because the man gave him ugly looks, and he recalled pushing another man in a crowded bus who got too close. Mr. AA. said drinking contributed to his actions and that he was old enough to know not to put his hands on others, that it had caused too much trouble for him. He acknowledged that alcohol gave him a bad attitude and that he needed to continue accepting medication. After he was seen by the hospital committee, his discharge to a supervised residence with an AOT order for injectable antipsychotic medication was approved.

10.4.2 Comment

Mr. AA. could be involuntarily admitted to hospital because, in view of his history, he was judged to be a risk to others when drinking and muttering threats. He could be retained involuntarily past the expiration of his initial commitment because he was seen as a risk in the community when he was without supervision. His treatment team needed time to find community supports that were appropriate for him.

Discharge planning is guided by obligations to maximize the chances that the patient and others will be safe and, at the same time, to offer the least restrictive setting. It requires assessment for risk of violence and suicide and for inability to meet basic needs, as well as risk management. Mr. AA.'s individual risk factors for violence were excess drinking, paranoid delusions about people of a different ethnic background, and a history of violent crime. Risk management for him was supervision and support from his ICM and from a supervised residence and an AOT order.

10.5 RISK FACTORS FOR VIOLENCE

10.5.1 Comparing former patients to their neighbors

A landmark study (Steadman et al., 1998) compared the prevalence of violence in about 1,000 men and women ages 18–40 who were recently discharged from acute psychiatric inpatient treatment to the prevalence of violence among their neighbors of the same age range. Choosing a control group of the same age range and socioeconomic status is important because, in a US survey of more than 10,000 adults (Swanson et al., 1990), rates of self-reported violent behavior vary with demographic variables. Rates are higher among younger people, men, and people who are poor.

To recruit for the Steadman study, people who had been hospitalized up to 21 days were approached a few days after hospital discharge and invited to participate. Violence was detected by self-report as well as by reports from police and a collateral informant. Of the former patient group, 39% were diagnosed with depression, 17% with schizophrenia, and 13% with bipolar disorder. These diagnoses were designated "major mental illness." Over a year of follow-up, there was no significant difference in the prevalence of violent behavior between the group of people with major mental illness without comorbid substance abuse and neighborhood controls without substance abuse. Active substance abuse increased the risk of violence in both major mental illness and control groups. Of the group with only major mental illness, 18% committed at least one violent act in a year, but 31% of those with comorbid substance abuse did so, a significant difference.

10.5.2 Diagnosis and prevalence of violence

Violence prevalence did not differ between the major mental illness group and controls, but is there a difference when diagnoses are separated out? In the large US survey noted above (Swanson et al., 1990), the prevalence of self-reported violence in community residents with no psychiatric disorder was 2%. It was 21% in those with substance abuse. Again, substance abuse increased violence risk. A diagnosis of an anxiety disorder alone was not associated with increased violence risk. A diagnosis of affective disorder alone was associated with a 3.4% prevalence of violence. A schizophrenia spectrum illness diagnosis alone was associated with an 8% rate. However, in the group with schizophrenia spectrum illness, almost a third had comorbid substance abuse. Substance abuse increased the risk of violence.

In New Zealand, investigators (Arseneault et al., 2000) followed 94% of people born in one city in a 12-month period, 961 in total. At age 21, subjects were interviewed to obtain diagnoses. Violent behavior in the prior year was measured with self-report and review of official conviction records. People with depressive and anxiety disorders were no more likely than people with without psychiatric disorders to be violent after controlling for substance abuse. Compared to people with no disorder, those with alcohol abuse were 1.9 times more likely to be violent, those with marijuana dependence were 3.8 times more likely, and those with schizophrenia spectrum illness were 2.5 times more likely. The number of subjects with mania was too small to draw conclusions. Comorbid substance abuse more than doubled the risk for violence in people with schizophrenia and related disorders. In the absence of substance abuse, violence in the group with schizophrenia spectrum disorders was related to a history of conduct disorder and excessive perceptions of risk (paranoia). However, only a small part (9.6%) of the risk of violence for the entire group of 961 people could be attributed to schizophrenia spectrum disorder.

Similarly, an Israeli epidemiologic study of 2,678 adults ages 24–33 (Stueve & Link, 1997) found that adults diagnosed with anxiety disorders or depression without psychosis had the same rate of self-reported physical fighting in the previous 5 years as adults with no psychiatric disorder, which was 7%. Adults with psychosis or bipolar disorder without comorbidity had higher rates (20.7%) in the previous 5 years. Comorbid substance abuse increased the rate to 39.3% in 5 years, and comorbid antisocial personality disorder, with or without substance abuse, increased the rate to 93.4%.

A 2022 analysis (Whiting et al.) of all studies available at the time concluded that a diagnosis of schizophrenia spectrum disorder alone increased the risk for violent behavior by about three times. With substance abuse comorbidity, the risk is increased about 10 times. This review took into account high-quality investigations newly available at the time that used national databases for diagnosis and criminal records to detect violent behavior.

The literature on bipolar disorder and violence is limited. One large study (Fazel et al., 2010a, 2010b) searched Swedish nationwide registries for records of hospital discharges and of convictions for violent crime. They compared 3,743 individuals discharged with diagnoses of bipolar disorder to general population controls. The increase in risk for patients with bipolar disorder alone was small (odds ratio [OR], 1.3). That is, the odds of conviction for violent crime were only slightly greater than the odds for the general population. For patients with comorbid substance abuse, the risk was greater (OR, 6.4).

10.5.3 Symptoms and violence

In surveys of the general population (Coid et al., 2016), paranoid ideation was associated with violence. Investigators pooled data from seven population surveys in Great Britain to obtain data on 23,444 adults. Paranoid ideation was associated with self-report of physical fighting or assault after controlling for demographic factors and substance abuse. A relationship they detected between probable psychosis and violence was explained by paranoia.

In an analysis of data (Ullrich et al., 2014) from the study described above of adults discharged from an acute psychiatric hospitalization (Steadman et al., 1998), paranoid, bizarre, and grandiose delusions detected in one evaluation were associated with violent behavior in the same evaluation period. (The people studied were a mixed diagnostic group.) All but grandiose delusions were associated with anger. After controlling for anger, the associations with violence were no longer significant. That is, anger was driving much of the relationship.

Studies on command auditory hallucinations are heterogenous in their methods and goals and inconsistent in results. One study of long-stay inpatients with chronic schizophrenia (Cheung et al., 1997) found no association between command hallucinations and violence. Another study (McNeil et al., 2000) of a group of inpatients with varied diagnoses found a relationship, but only in the context of other psychotic symptoms. A summary of the available literature

(Braham et al., 2004) concluded that some people will act on hallucinations, but hallucinations alone are not enough to produce action. Action seems to depend on mediating variables such as beliefs about the hallucinated voice and the instructions it gives.

10.5.4 Lack of treatment and violence

In a Swedish pharmacoepidemiologic study (Fazel et al., 2014), lack of treatment was related to violence. Using nationwide registries, investigators identified 82,647 people who were prescribed antipsychotics or mood stabilizers. They also noted their diagnoses and criminal histories. When people with diagnoses of bipolar disorder or schizophrenia were prescribed antipsychotic drugs or mood stabilizers, they were less likely to be convicted for violent crimes than when they were not prescribed. Violent crime was 45% less likely on antipsychotics. It was 24% less likely on mood stabilizers, but only for people with bipolar disorder. Rates of violent crime decreased when an antipsychotic was added to a mood stabilizer but not when a mood stabilizer was added to an antipsychotic drug.

10.5.5 A summary

A review (Lagerberg et al., 2025) of recent publications that reported on studies of people with psychotic illnesses (including schizophrenia-spectrum, schizotypal disorder, bipolar disorder, and affective psychosis but excluding drug-induced psychosis) identified risk factors discovered in at least two independent groups of subjects. Criminal history was associated with the greatest risk of violence, followed by substance abuse. Other risk factors were paranoia, hostility, recent violent victimization, a history of parental violent crime, comorbid personality disorder, number of past hospitalizations, male gender, youth, and a history of self-harm. A diagnosis of schizophrenia was associated with more risk compared to other diagnoses. Treatment with antipsychotic medication was associated with less risk.

REFERENCES

Arseneault, L., Moffit, T. E., Caspi, A. S., Taylor, P. J., & Silva, P. A. (2000). Mental disorders and violence in a total birth cohort: Results from the Dunedin Study. *Archives of General Psychiatry* 57:979–986.

Braham, L. G., Trower, P., & Birchwood, M. (2004). Acting on command hallucinations and dangerous behavior: A critique of the major findings in the last decade. *Clinical Psychology Review* 24(5):513–528.

Cheung, P., Schweitzer, I., Crowley, K., & Tuckwell, V. (1997). Violence in schizophrenia: Role of hallucinations and delusions. *Schizophrenia Research* 26:181–190.

Coid, J. W., Ullriochj, S., Bebbington, P., Fazel, S., & Keers, R. (2016). Paranoid ideation and violence: Meta-analysis of individual subject data of 7 population surveys. *Schizophrenia Bulletin* 42:907–915.

Fazel, S., Lichtenstein, P., Frisell, T., Grann, M., Goodwin, G. M., & Langstrom, N. (2010a). Bipolar disorders and violent crime: new evidence from population-based longitudinal studies and systematic review. *Archives of General Psychiatry* 67:931–938.

Fazel, S., Lichtenstein, P., Frisell, T., Grann, M., Goodwin, G. M., & Langstrom, N. (2010b). Bipolar disorders and violent crime: Time at risk reanalysis. *Archives of General Psychiatry* 67:1325–1326.

Fazel, S., Zetterqvist, J., Larsson, H., Langstrom, N., & Lichtenstein, P. (2014). Antipsychotics, mood stabilizers, and risk of violent crime. *Lancet* 384:1206–1214.

Lagerberg, T., Lambe, S., Paulino, A., Yu, R., & Fazel, S. (2025). Systematic review of risk factors for violence in psychosis: A 10-year update. *British Journal of Psychiatry* 226(2):100–107.

McNeil, D. E., Eisner, J. P., & Binder, R. L. (2000). The relationship between command hallucinations and violence. *Psychiatric Services* 51(10):1288–1292.

Steadman, H. J., Mulvey, E. D., Monahan, J., Robbins, P. C. Appelbaum, P. S., Grissao, T., . . . & Silver, E. (1998). Violence by people discharged from acute psychiatric inpatient facilities and by others in the same neighborhoods. *Archives of General Psychiatry* 55:393–401.

Stueve, A., & Link, B. (1997). Violence and psychiatric disorders: Results from an epidemiologic study of young adults in Israel. *Psychiatric Quarterly* 68:327–342.

Swanson, J. W., Holzer, C. E., Ganju, V. K., & Jono, R. T. (1990). Violence and psychiatric disorder in the community. *Hospital and Community Psychiatry* 41:761–770.

Ullrich, S., Keers, R., & Coid, J. W. (2014). Delusions, anger, and serious violence: New findings from the MacArthur Risk Assessment Study. *Schizophrenia Bulletin* 40:1174–1181.

Whiting, D., Gulati, G., Geddes, J. R., & Fazel, S. (2022). Association of schizophrenia-spectrum disorders and violence perpetration I adults and adolescents from 15 countries: A systematic review and meta-analysis. *JAMA Psychiatry* 79(2):120–132.

11

OUTPATIENT COMMITMENT

This chapter outlines and illustrates, through four cases, criteria and procedures for obtaining outpatient commitment as well as the limitations of this intervention. Outpatient commitment is court-ordered community treatment for patients whose nonadherence with medications has led to hospitalization, incarceration, or violence. It is a form of risk management that involves some coercion.

11.1 CASE BB: NOT A CANDIDATE

11.1.1 Case

Mr. BB. was a man in his 40s admitted to a state psychiatric hospital after he was found not fit to proceed and his charges were dropped. His alleged crime was violating an order of protection obtained by a woman who lived in his residence.

Interview

Mr. BB. was dressed in sweatpants and a tee shirt and on crutches. He had a cast on his leg, sutures in one elbow, and a red and swollen eye, all he explained, the outcome of a fight that occurred in jail. His psychiatrist also noticed tissue paper stuffed into both ears.

When asked, "Why are you here?" Mr. BB. said, "It's a mix up. Things happen and I'm here. Certain things are classified. Don't write them down. They should not be written in the computer." He said he had studied psychology and psychiatry, that he was being persecuted for righteousness' sake, and that when you're blessed certain things happen. He did not deny or confirm that he was a prophet, and, when asked if he heard the voice of God, said he would not get into that. And the tissue paper? It was too noisy in jail. He denied he had never been hospitalized for psychiatric illness or taken mental health medication.

History

Mr. BB. had never been arrested before. His only previous psychiatric admissions were for treatment of alcohol abuse, the most recent 10 years earlier.

Course of treatment

Mr. BB. was seen by an orthopedic surgeon at a local general hospital who found fractures in bones in his foot and reapplied a cast. On the ward, he followed the routine, kept himself clean and neat, and harassed nobody.

The treatment team social worker recognized the address he gave as a supervised residence for psychiatrically ill adults. That, his Supplemental Security Income (SSI) benefits, and his intake interview led his psychiatrist to ask him to consider taking medication. He was thankful for treatment of his broken foot but declared that he did not need medication and that there was nothing psychiatrically wrong with him.

Mr. BB. refused to sign consent to allow the social worker to speak with staff at his residence although she told him that she had to verify that he had a place to live before he could be discharged. "You should worry about yourself," he told her. He was not worried about himself; God would care for him. Tissue paper was still stuffed in his ears, which raised the suspicion he was hallucinating. His litigiousness was demonstrated by the pile of legal documents he brandished, part of his suit against a local medical clinic.

Although he said he would refuse medications, when a nurse offered it, he accepted an antipsychotic drug. With treatment he was less intense and less hostile but still paranoid. Another antipsychotic drug was no more effective.

He never agreed to release information to his residence, but an employee there was free to share information with his treatment team. The employee told the ward social worker that Mr. BB. was welcome to return. Mr. BB. basically did not present problems, she said, though he did not attend outpatient clinic. His legal problems began with a friendship with a female resident. When she no longer wanted contact with him, he would not back off but continued to knock on her door several times a day. The resident then felt compelled to obtain an order of protection.

Mr. BB. wanted to leave the hospital and return to his residence, where he planned to help out fellow tenants, pursue his lawsuit, volunteer at his church, and avoid the woman who had an order of protection against him. When asked what he thought of his medication, he replied, "No comment." He said that he did not have a psychiatric problem but would do what he had to do while in the hospital. And afterward? He had to think about whether he would take medication after discharge.

Mr. BB. was discharged back to his residence without an outpatient commitment order.

11.1.2 Comment

Mr. BB. was not a suitable candidate for outpatient commitment. His psychiatrist could not testify that for him treatment noncompliance led to multiple recent incarcerations or hospitalizations, or that without treatment he would pose a risk of serious harm to himself or to others.

On the ward, he was not a threat to others, and he cared for himself. His past performance outside the hospital had been similar, even though he did not attend a clinic or take psychotropic medication. For several years he had maintained himself in a community residence. He was welcome to return. He had no history of violent crime.

11.1.3 Criteria

Court-ordered community treatment goes by different names including *outpatient commitment, community treatment orders, civil commitment*, and *compulsory* or *mandatory outpatient commitment* (Segal, 2022). In the US state where Mr. BB. was hospitalized, it was called *assisted outpatient treatment* (AOT). People eligible for AOT in that state are older than 18 years and suffer from a mental illness. They must have a history of noncompliance with treatment and be unlikely to accept treatment voluntarily in the future due to mental illness.

It is a form of coercive risk management. Criteria include a likelihood of benefit and a level of risk without intervention. Eligible patients must be unlikely to survive safely in the community without supervision. They must need AOT to prevent deterioration or relapse that would likely result in serious harm to the patient or to other people.

In addition, treatment noncompliance must have led to hospitalization or incarceration at least twice in the past 36 months, or noncompliance must have led to one or more serious acts of, threats of, or attempts at serious physical violence toward self or others within the past 48 months (Behnke et al., 2003).

REFERENCES

Behnke, S. H., Perlin, M. L., & Bernstein, M. (2003). *The Essentials of New York Mental Health Law: A Straightforward Guide for Clinicians of All Disciplines*. New York: Norton, pp. 98–100.

Segal, S. P. (2022). Protecting health and safety with needed-treatment: The effectiveness of outpatient commitment. *Psychiatric Quarterly* 93(1):55–79.

11.2 CASE CC: JUST A MUSICIAN TRYING TO MAKE IT

11.2.1 Case

Mr. CC. was in his 30s when he was admitted to a state psychiatric hospital after being charged with harassment and found not fit to stand trial. His charges, which were related to allegedly making many threatening phone calls to a concert venue owner, were dropped.

Interview

Mr. CC. was in dirty clothes, unshaved and smelly. He remained polite while he excitedly shared his plans for his rap music career: to tour with a famous rapper, perform at major venues, and make millions of dollars. When his psychiatrist expressed skepticism, he pulled out pages covered with rap lyrics to demonstrate evidence of his superior talent. He had no idea why he was sent to the hospital and denied ever experiencing auditory hallucinations.

Mr. CC. reported that in high school he performed as a rapper and in college he studied music recording. Subsequent years were rootless and centered on his drive to become a star. He moved to a distant state where he harassed concert venue bookers and owners. At times he was held in psychiatric hospitals for treatment, but usually his stays were short because he was not considered dangerous. Once he was kept longer, for about 2 months. At times he lived in a rooming house where his landlord was his Supplemental Security Income (SSI) payee, but he was dissatisfied with the amount of spending money the landlord gave him. At times he lived on the streets.

After 9 years, he moved to another part of the country where he lived in a rented room, was his own payee, and again badgered concert venues in his quest to promote his career. Mr. CC. kept on moving from one region of the country to another.

History

When examiners found him unfit, they noted signs and symptoms of a psychotic illness including auditory hallucinations, disconnected thinking, and incredible statements such that he had fathered 20 children.

Mr. CC.'s parents appeared at the hospital in person within a day or two after their son supplied their phone number. His father recalled a distant afternoon when he discovered his teenaged son wrapped in gauze bandages and going on about strange ideas. Mr. CC. said voices were talking to him from fiber optic cables overhead. His father immediately drove him to a local psychiatric hospital, where his son was admitted and treated for a few weeks. This was an extended stay compared to the 3–7 days that were typical of his later hospitalizations, probably because, at a retention hearing, the younger Mr. CC. agreed he should stay for a while. According to his parents, this was the only time their son was aware that he had a psychiatric problem.

For several months in his heathier days, many years ago, Mr. CC. performed, but only occasionally and at open-microphone nights on small local stages. He had not performed for an audience for at least 20 years, but had single-mindedly pursued a music career. This fixation led to numerous arrests and one incarceration of several months for harassment, but, as far as they knew, no arrests for violent crimes.

The parents said their son was not tuned in to his problem. He disagreed when they suggested he had a mental illness, did not renew psychiatrists' prescriptions, and did not attend outpatient clinics. He accepted a supervised residence for adults with serious mental illness only once, early in his illness, and stayed not more than a day or two. Instead, he chose homeless shelters or flophouses—multiple flophouses because he was evicted from one after another.

His parents complained that, except for promoting his nonexistent music career, he lacked initiative. He shunned hard work, preferred to stay in bed, and, without supervision, did not keep his body or his room clean.

Their son was at his best for a period of a couple of years, starting a few years before his current admission, when hospital doctors in another state obtained an outpatient commitment order. He was followed by an assertive community treatment (ACT) team and accepted court-ordered long-acting intramuscular medication. At his best he was able to socialize with his family. This time came to an end when he was again evicted and moved to another state where his outpatient commitment order was not binding.

Course of treatment

Because the antipsychotic drug Mr. CC. accepted in jail and on the ward seemed ineffective, he was given a trial of clozapine. Over the course of his hospital stay he maintained that he was wasting his time, time that should be spent furthering his career. "How long do I have to stay?" he asked. "I'll quit calling those guys. I'm just a musician trying to make it."

Progress was slow. He disclosed multiple implausible ideas such that he had had a romantic relationship with a female pop star that resulted in multiple children. Mr. CC. was unhappy in the hospital because he believed he was pushed to do too much. He had no interest in the patient work program or in performing in a ward talent show. Ward attendants had to encourage him to shower, shave, change clothes, and keep his personal area tidy. All the while, he lobbied for discharge as soon as possible.

At the suggestion of discharge to a residence or group home, he asked if he would have to stay. He planned to move on to a distant part of the country to promote his music. His parents traveled many miles from their home to visit every weekend and saw no change in their son. They did not mention his obvious 10-pound weight gain.

11.2.2 Comment

As much as they cared about their son, his parents could not keep Mr. CC. settled. Neither could supervised housing. Jails and psychiatric hospitals could keep him tied down, but for no more than a few months. Mostly he dodged both jail and psychiatric hospitals because he was not seen as dangerous. His psychiatrist was hopeful that a trial of clozapine would decrease his fixation on a musical career and therefore help him to consider staying in one place and reestablishing a close relationship with his family, but it did not.

His parents remembered the most stable years he had were the 2 he spent in another area of the country with an ACT team and a court order for intramuscular medication. The ACT team gave him intensive supervision and monitoring and the court order added coercion. His court order was limited to the state he left, and he was not eligible for another order in the state where he was treated. By moving again, he once again dodged treatment and stability.

11.3 CASE DD: SENT BY JESUS

11.3.1 Case

Ms. DD. was a woman in her 40s who was admitted to a state psychiatric hospital after being found not fit to proceed and her charges dropped. She had allegedly violated an order of protection when she interrupted a movie screening at a local theater by shouting obscenities and refusing to leave.

Interview

Ms. DD. sat straight-backed, calmly holding her hands in her lap. She was a neat woman, unadorned by jewelry, makeup, or fancy dress. She held her psychiatrist's gaze as she answered questions, sometimes tilting her chin up to look down at the doctor as she spoke. Her replies were unhesitating and confident.

She explained that she had been hearing the voices of Jesus and angels for many years. Jesus sent her to the movie theater to be a messenger to His people. His message was that pornography is a sin. Many movies playing at the theater were called love stories but were in reality nothing more than pornography. Also, she wanted to proclaim Jesus's laws, which forbid eating certain fruits and vegetables and favored others. She was angry that the theater and its manager showed no interest in the words of Our Lord.

Ms. DD. also a message for the hospital where she had been treated previously. They told her she had a mental problem. She did not have any mental problem. In addition, she had a message for the psychiatrist interviewing her. She would not be taking medication. Though she took it before, it was only because she was told that if she did not, she would not leave the hospital. After discharge, she threw it in the garbage. She never took medication after discharge.

History from cinema manager

Mr. W. said that he ran a small local theater that catered to families with children. It never showed sexy movies. He complained that, for the past few years, Ms. DD. would disrupt movie screenings every week. She would stand close to the screen and yell and scream about pornography and what Mr. W. called "nonsense about food." Once Ms. DD. kicked the manager as he tried to lead her out the door. Mr. W. finally sought and obtained an order of protection for himself and his theater after Ms. DD. slapped a woman who asked her sit down and keep quiet.

The criminal justice system and the psychiatric service of the local hospital delivered only short-term, intermittent relief. At least five times in the previous 3 years Ms. DD. had been arrested for violating an order of protection and, directly from jail, transferred to the local hospital. She would be absent from the theater for several weeks but reliably returned to ruining her neighbors' night out at the movies.

History from records

For many years Ms. DD. had attended an outpatient clinic in her neighborhood. Psychiatrists at the clinic wrote that she would typically be admitted to hospital because she disrupted a local movie theater after months of refusing medication. She had been hospitalized for treatment of psychiatric illness more than 10 times over the previous 5 years, with 4 of those admissions in the previous 24 months. Prior to one admission, she forcefully slapped her therapist, saying she was commanded to do so by a heavenly angel. During this hospital stay, Ms. DD. was treated with a long-acting injectable antipsychotic. With treatment, her religious delusions eased, her behavior changed, and she gained some insight.

Ms. DD. was discharged to a different clinic on a monthly antipsychotic injection and a mood stabilizer. Clinic notes revealed that, soon after she was discharged, she no longer brought fruits and vegetables to distribute to clinic staff. She explained that her ideas about food were part of her illness that she had given up for good. In a month, she complained of pain where she was given injections and asked to take pills instead, so she was prescribed pills instead of injections. In 3 months, she was back to toting produce to the clinic and lecturing about heavenly dietary laws. In a few months, her clinic attendance became erratic. Nine months after discharge, she was arrested.

Course of treatment

On the ward, Ms. DD. was true to her word in that she refused every dose of antipsychotic that was offered to her. Rather than participate in ward groups or activities, she spent hours praying loudly on her knees at the end of an isolated corridor. If other patients approached she would berate them for what she saw as incorrect diets and immodest choice of dress. They learned to steer clear of her.

Her psychiatrist explained the risks and benefits of antipsychotic medication and that she had an illness. A court application for permission to give intramuscular medication over her objection was granted. Within a few weeks of her second monthly injection she had stopped praying loudly and chastising others. Her comments in ward groups were logical and relevant. Rather than haughty and impassioned, she became pleasant and shy. She denied hearing the voices of Jesus and angels and said she did not want to be looking for trouble so she would stay away from the movie theater.

Her psychiatrist also made an application to court for assisted outpatient treatment (AOT). Part of the application was an individualized treatment plan that included regular clinic appointments and monthly injections of the antipsychotic drug she had taken on the ward. A case manager would monitor Ms. HH's needs, access to services, and adherence. Ms. DD. agreed to the plan and a judge agreed to an AOT order. She was discharged to the home she shared with a family member.

11.3.2 A good candidate

Ms. DD. was a good candidate for court-ordered outpatient treatment. She had a well-documented history of nonadherence to treatment and, due to mental illness, was unlikely to accept treatment voluntarily in the future. She certainly met the criteria for at least two incarcerations or hospital admissions due to noncompliance in the previous 36 months. Because she had shown a clear positive response to antipsychotic medication in the hospital, she was likely to benefit from outpatient treatment. Ms. DD. needed AOT to prevent relapse, which would likely result in harm to patrons of Mr. W.'s cinema.

11.3.3 AOT treatment plans

Ms. DD.'s AOT order was based on a treatment plan tailored to her needs. In testimony, her psychiatrist was required to argue why all elements of the treatment plan were necessary for this particular patient and why the plan was the least restrictive possible. As required by the law of her state, the plan included enhanced services, that is, case management services or an assertive community treatment (ACT) team. When plans include medication, the particular medication and its administration schedule must be specified. Plans can include other categories of services, such as supervised housing or substance abuse treatment with urine or blood testing for illicit substances.

If Ms. DD. were to fail to comply with treatment, those treating her as an outpatient were required to solicit compliance. If these efforts were to fail and a physician decided she met criteria for involuntary admission, he or she could direct police or a sheriff to transport her to a hospital for examination (Behnke et al., 2003).

11.3.4 Patient outcomes with AOT

To assess the effectiveness of AOT in New York state, Swartz and colleagues (2010) compared patient outcomes before and after an AOT order. They searched Medicaid and state hospital records for 3,576 individuals with AOT orders. During the first 6 months with an order, the likelihood of hospitalization was decreased significantly, by 25%, compared to before AOT. After 12 months, if the order was renewed, the likelihood of hospitalization was decreased further. A measure of medication compliance increased by almost 50% in the first 6-month period and by almost 90% in the following 6 months.

Investigators also compared people with ACT teams but not an AOT order to people with both. Patients who had both ACT teams and an AOT order had significantly less risk of hospitalization during any 6 months after the first 6 months of AOT compared to patients with ACT teams alone, with an odds ratio of .43. This is evidence that AOT's impact on hospitalization risk is not only due to the increased services offered by an ACT team. The authors cautioned that these findings may not hold in states with less well-funded mental health and outpatient commitment programs.

Another study (Phelan et al., 2010) followed 76 people with recent AOT orders and108 people without AOT orders for 1 year. All subjects were attending the same New York state outpatient clinic. Suicide risk and self-reported violent behavior were significantly lower in the group with AOT, while psychotic symptoms and quality of life were not significantly different. The odds of serious violent behavior during 12 months of follow-up were more than four times larger in the group without AOT compared to the group with AOT.

REFERENCES

Behnke, S. H., Perlin, M. L., & Bernstein, M. (2003). *The Essentials of New York Mental Health Law: A Straightforward Guide for Clinicians of All Disciplines.* New York: Norton, pp. 98–100.

Phelan, J. C., Sinkewicz, M., Castille, D. M., Huz, S., & Link, B. G. (2010). Effectiveness and outcomes of assisted outpatient treatment in New York State. *Psychiatric Services* 61(2):137–143.

Swartz, M. S., Wilder, C. M., Swanson, J. W., Van Dorn, R. A., Robbins, P. C., Steadman, H. J., . . . & Monahan, J. (2010). Assessing outcomes for consumers in New York's assisted outpatient treatment program. *Psychiatric Services* 61(10):976–981.

11.4 CASE EE: MANY TRIALS OF OUTPATIENT COMMITMENT

11.4.1 Case

Ms. EE. was a woman in her 40s who was charged with assault, found not fit to stand trial, and admitted to a state psychiatric hospital for restoration of fitness. Her alleged offense was an assault on a nurse in a community hospital where police had transported her at the request of her assertive community treatment (ACT) team because she was 2 months overdue for the long-acting antipsychotic injection that was part of her assisted outpatient treatment (AOT) plan.

Course of treatment

In her first few weeks in the state hospital, Ms. EE. was intensely and persistently angry and aggressive. Fights erupted all around her as she went about her day provoking other patients. After she consistently accepted a long-acting injectable antipsychotic drug, the ward returned to its mostly peaceful state.

Interview

Ms. EE. was a lively, engaging woman who easily smiled and laughed when she joined her treatment team around a conference room table. "You've become a different person," her psychiatrist said.

Ms. EE.: I had an attitude change. I tried to cooperate. Before I didn't want to be in the hospital; I'd rather be at school or work.
Psychiatrist: What about the medication you're taking? What do you think of it?
Ms. EE.: It's a nice medication, but I don't know if it helped me.
Psychiatrist: You were very irritable.

Ward staff chimed in that she was so much better.

Ms. EE.: I'm more laid back, but I'm not sure if it was bipolar or that I just didn't want to be in the hospital.
Psychiatrist: I think you're bipolar. You've been getting nowhere. You keep getting into hospitals. If you keep taking medication, you could turn your life around. You could train to become a peer counselor.

Ms. EE. laughed and said that she would hang in there. "I have a nice family," she said, "I used to have a job working in a park. I pay attention to the attendants. They clock in and clock out. I don't pay attention to the patients."

History

Ms. EE.'s hospitalizations for psychiatric illness began when she was a teenager, with many, many admissions to community hospitals and several to state hospitals over the course of her life. Over the years, psychiatrists discharged her with an AOT order at least four times.

In her 30s, Ms. EE. was admitted to a community hospital after she hit a social service worker. From the community hospital she was transferred to a state hospital where she also hit and kicked employees. With court-ordered medication she eventually became less manic and was discharged to her family home with an AOT order.

A few years later, she was admitted to another community hospital where she hit staff and patients. She was successfully treated over objection and discharged but was soon arrested for violating an order of protection brought by a family member and sent to jail. After being found not fit to stand trial, she was sent to a state hospital, treated, and discharged to a state clinic with an AOT order.

When seen in the clinic weeks later she was not manic but calmly related that a transmitter installed in her head made her hear the voice of a former high school teacher. After a few months attending clinic appointments, she disappeared. She was hospitalized again and then returned to clinic where she complained of feeling without spirits and uninterested in doing anything. At this time she was only accepting a low dose of quetiapine but also using methamphetamine. Ms. EE. continued attending clinic for about a year.

After another few years and a few community hospitalizations, she was discharged from a state hospital with an AOT order. Within a few weeks her family called her ACT team because she was not sleeping, kept her family up at night playing loud music, and was seen urinating and defecating behind bushes in her neighborhood. The ACT team took her to a community hospital that transferred her to a state hospital. After treatment over objection, Ms. EE. was discharged with an AOT order, but, at this point, finding an ACT team was difficult because a number of ACT teams remembered and refused her.

Two years later, a family member called police because Ms. EE. was screaming and threatening an elderly aunt. Police transported Ms. EE. to a community hospital. On the ward, she assaulted another patient, was treated over objection, and then transferred to a state hospital. The state facility again obtained an AOT order. On discharge, Ms. EE. was polite and cooperative and said she understood that if she did not show up for a monthly injection she could be readmitted.

She met with her ACT team regularly for several months but then became erratic. Two months passed without contact with the team and without a long-acting antipsychotic injection. Police took her to a local community hospital where she was again manic and refusing medication and where, soon after a judge ordered treatment over objection, she attacked a nurse.

In jail, she refused psychotropic medication. When mental health workers stopped by her cell she said she only wanted to talk about getting bailed out, not about medication. But she was not bailed out. From jail she was sent to the state hospital where her psychiatrist told her that if she kept taking medication she could turn her life around.

11.4.2 Comment

Ms. EE.'s manic symptoms responded well to medication—so well, it was as if she became a different person. But she was still the woman who, after many years of hospitalizations and incarcerations, was not sure she had a severe psychiatric illness or that medication helped her. She distanced herself from the other patients on her ward and identified with the staff. The consequences of her illness could have been very different if she were consistently taking medication and engaged in treatment.

She was not held in hospitals against her will once her mania remitted. To meet the challenge of keeping her in treatment after discharge, psychiatrists employed coercive measures. They obtained AOT orders along with ICMs and ACT teams. AOT and treatment over objection resulted in compliance with treatment and remission of symptoms, but only temporarily.

Her AOT team waited 2 months after Ms. EE. was due for her injection to request transport to an emergency room. If she were sent earlier, before she became manic, the course of events might have been different. By law, though, a physician had to decide she met criteria for involuntary admission before he or she could direct police or a sheriff to transport her to a hospital for examination (Behnke et al., 2003).

Over many years, the cost of her illness and its treatment was steep for Ms. EE., her family, and hospital staff. For some hospital staff, such as the community hospital nurse whom she assaulted, the cost was too high. The nurse chose to press charges against Ms. EE., thus turning to the criminal justice system for relief. Ms. EE. was contained in jail but, because she refused, not treated in jail.

REFERENCE

Behnke, S. H., Perlin, M. L., & Bernstein, M. (2003). *The Essentials of New York Mental Health Law: A Straightforward Guide for Clinicians of All Disciplines*. New York: Norton, pp. 98–100.

12

INTERSECTION WITH THE CRIMINAL JUSTICE SYSTEM

People in the public psychiatry system are often arrested and sometimes incarcerated, as detailed in this chapter. The criminal justice system can provide coercion or risk management, as illustrated in the case of a patient on parole and the case of a man who screened for admission to an alternatives to incarceration program. Additional cases describe the lives and treatment of 2 men who were frequently incarcerated. One seemed to suffer from both schizophrenia and anti-social personality disorder.

12.1 CASE FF: A MAN ON PAROLE

12.1.1 Case

Mr. FF. was a man in his 40s who was admitted directly to a state psychiatric hospital on the day of his release from prison.

Interview

Mr. FF. was a trim and clean man dressed in his prison-issued shirt and pants; he said he was feeling splendid. His attention darted off in all directions, but, with some effort, his psychiatrist could redirect him and gather information. "My main projective is to live a positive, enthusiastic life," he said. He had no idea why he was sent to the hospital. He volunteered that he had no delusions or hallucinations. When asked, he denied that he was very wealthy, that he had a special relationship to God, special powers and abilities, or that he thought other people in prison wanted to hurt him.

Mr. FF. said that after his most recent release from prison, he immediately scuttled his discharge plan and moved into his mother's home, his go-to home when he was not in prison or jail. Though he reported to his parole officer as required, sought employment, and participated in group therapy at the Fortune Society, all with a goal to, as he put it, motivate, accumulate, and elevate in life, he failed to report to his outpatient clinic and take psychotropic medication. He said it made him sick to his stomach.

History

Prison records documented that Mr. FF.'s psychiatric treatment began when he was a young man and continued for the majority of the previous 20 years, mostly coincident with the years he spent in prison.

His most recent prison bid began several years earlier, when he was convicted of a dangerous felony. After most of his sentence was complete, he was released on parole to a state hospital, treated, and discharged to a supervised residence. As he reported in his admitting interview, he violated the terms of his parole by walking out of his supervised residence and discontinuing psychiatric treatment. He was, therefore, reincarcerated.

Prison psychiatrists who treated him before he finished his sentence wrote that he had grandiose delusions and behavior problems in that he was loud, disruptive, and threatening. Psychiatrists prescribed and nurses offered medication, but he rarely took it.

Course of treatment

Mr. FF. sat at the head of a long table in a conference room as his treatment team members sat along each side. He watched and listened intently, identifying and addressing each person individually. He shared his plans to motivate, accumulate, and elevate. Then his psychiatrist presented him with a diagnosis—bipolar disorder—and explained the risks and benefits of proposed treatment with a mood stabilizer. His response was to insist he was not mentally ill, to complain he was being abused, and to state that he would refuse. But, to the psychiatrist's surprise and relief, when nurses offered divalproex, he took it.

Mr. FF. was on parole for life. Just as at his last psychiatric hospitalization, one condition of his parole was to accept psychiatric treatment after discharge. So, soon after Mr. FF. arrived, his parole officer came to the hospital to check on his charge and meet his treatment team. He requested and got regular, open communication and collaborative discharge planning.

While slowly and gradually increasing his dose of mood stabilizer, the doctor did not detect side effects and Mr. FF. did not report them. He was quick to anger but kept his hands to himself; he was ingratiating with staff but domineering with other patients. In groups, he took center stage to lecture other patients on how they should behave better. While he was mostly logical he relied heavily on a few vague phrases repeated over and over. After a few weeks he gave up his prison uniform.

Over time, it became clear that divalproex did little for him. Staff from a complaint line called to report that he was calling many, many times; not threatening, but harassing, leaving rambling and illogical messages. When offered risperidone, he accepted. After a few weeks he slowed down. He no longer dominated all group discussions, nor did he barrage the telephone complaint phone line.

By this time his discharge process was moving along. Mr. FF. was willing to accept living in a residence as long as he could visit his mother on weekends, but, after interviews at two residences, he was rejected by both. Disheartened, he asked for discharge to the on-grounds state residence.

Mr. FF. shared his plans for his future out of the hospital. He would stay focused, maintain employment, and help his mother. He would live a positive, enthusiastic life. He would be productive and stay out of trouble. He would attend clinic and, in his spare time, exercise, listen to music, and read books. And he promised he would not run off to live with his mother.

While he said he wanted to reward his team's trust in him, he also knew that, just like before, if he were to abscond he would violate the terms of his parole and return to prison. He acknowledged the sad truth of his life, that he had already spent too much time incarcerated. And he could say that, with medication, he was able to take his time and not talk so fast.

12.1.2 Comment

Mr. FF's parole officer and his psychiatric treatment team worked together to supervise him. They cooperated because both had an obligation to keep both this man and their community safe. The criminal justice system, represented by his parole officer, provided more leverage than would an assisted outpatient treatment (AOT) order. That leverage and cooperation would continue after discharge, but with outpatient clinic and residence staff.

No residence would accept Mr. FF. other than the hospital's own residence, likely because of his criminal history. In 2004, investigators (Way et al.) noted that a group of patients transferred to a civil hospital from a prison psychiatric hospital took one and a half times as long to be discharged as patients not admitted from prison hospitals, although the two groups of patients were comparable in diagnoses and functioning.

12.1.3 Specialty parole and probation

Mr. FF. had a parole officer whose caseload was limited to individuals with severe mental illness. Much like specialty probation officers, his parole officer had a smaller case load than traditional parole officers and had undergone sustained training in mental health. His parole officer was more focused on treatment than on punishment. A comparison of rates of arrest in groups of probationers with mental illness assigned to traditional versus specialty mental health probation discovered that the group in traditional probation was 2.68 times more likely to be arrested within 2 years than the specialty group.

12.1.4 Leverage

Cooperation with treatment as a condition of parole is a form of leverage or coercion. It is one of multiple types of leverage used with people with severe mental illness in the community. In the criminal justice system, leverage can take the form of treatment as a condition of probation or parole or as an alternative to incarceration. Leverage can consist of conditioning access to funds on treatment adherence, a strategy used by some money managers, people who hold and manage disability benefits. Housing programs may require participation in treatment or sobriety to obtain or continue in housing. Outpatient commitment or AOT is another form of leverage. Leverage is used significantly more often with younger patients and with those with more severe, disabling, and longer-term pathology, multiple hospitalizations, and intensive outpatient service use (Monahan et al., 2005).

REFERENCES

Monahan, J., Redlich, A. D., Swanson, J., Robbins, P. C., Appelbaum, P. S., Petrila, J. . . . & McNiel, D. E. (2005). Use of leverage to improve adherence to psychiatric treatment in the community. *Psychiatric Services* 56(1):37–44.

Skeem, J. L., Manchak, S., & Montoya, L. (2017). Comparing public safety outcomes for traditional probation vs. specialty mental health probation. *JAMA Psychiatry* 74(9):942–948.

Way, B. B., Smith, H., & Sawyer, D. (2004). Transfers to civil psychiatric inpatient services from a maximum security forensic hospital. *Behavioral Sciences and the Law* 22(2):253–259.

12.2 CASE GG: ALTERNATIVES TO INCARCERATION

12.2.1 Case

Mr. GG. was a man in his 40's who, upon referral by his outpatient psychiatrist, was admitted to the same state psychiatric hospital that had discharged him less than 2 years earlier.

Interview

On his admission interview, Mr. GG. related that although he was provided housing in the supervised residence on hospital grounds, he walked out and instead moved into a low-rent hotel, also known as a flophouse. For a year and a half he lived there, supporting himself with food stamps and his Social Security benefits. For a few weeks he held a low-wage hourly job, but lost it when his boss learned he came from a mental asylum.

All took a turn for the worse when another hotel resident threatened him with a knife. Mr. GG. pressed legal charges and then moved out. Because he believed the long-acting injectable antipsychotic injections he was getting at an outpatient clinic impaired his balance, slurred his speech, and made him sleepy and overweight, he quit accepting injections. There was absolutely no way he had a psychiatric problem, he said.

History

Mr. GG. graduated high school, then studied at an art school. The first of many psychiatric hospitalizations occurred in his 20s.

His previous admission to the same hospital began after he was charged with a misdemeanor assault on a stranger on the streets, for which he offered a bizarre explanation and was found not fit to stand trial. A psychiatrist tried at least four different antipsychotic drugs, including clozapine, but none was more effective than the long-acting injectable on which he was discharged. After an extended stay, Mr. GG. was discharged to the supervised residence on hospital grounds.

Mr. GG.'s outpatient psychiatrist had observed his patient on the snowy December streets close to the clinic buttonholing passersby and wearing a sign that read, "No soul thieves!" When seen in clinic he was smelly, dressed in a flimsy jacket, his sock reddened by blood oozing from a venous stasis ulcer. He began his visit with his psychiatrist by explaining that he was trying to warn the public about a secret organization that telepathically robbed people's souls, but abruptly interrupted himself to ask for food.

Course of treatment

Mr. GG. readily settled into life on the ward. With resumption of a long-acting injectable antipsychotic drug, he stopped spontaneously and excitedly telling others about soul robbers, but, if asked, claimed such a phenomena was possible. He stayed to himself, washed up, and ate well. His ulcers were cleaned and dressed. At a patient art show employees and patients lined up to buy his deftly drawn portraits and evocative landscapes. Mr. GG. was again discharged to the hospital's residence.

12.2.2 Two years later

Mr. GG. was arrested for an apparently inexplicable assault on a random person on the street. He was found not fit to stand trial and sent to a state hospital for restoration of fitness. After this was accomplished, he returned to jail, where he waited months for disposition of his case. About 2 years after he was discharged to a state hospital's on-grounds supervised residence, he was interviewed for acceptance into an alternatives to incarceration program.

Interview

Mr. GG. was animated and friendly and could speak logically, but only up to a point. When asked about his alleged crime, he said his arm was moved telepathically by someone else, someone who was working on stealing his soul. His mood was fine, and he denied hallucinations.

From the hospital on-grounds residence Mr. GG. found his way to a low-rent hotel, where he said his experience was fantastic. The place was clean, no drug addicts lived there, and a social service agency regularly sent a van to sit outside and offer free food. "At the hotel, you're not treated like you're from a mental institution," he said. He explained that being treated that way meant "they won't talk to you because they think they're better than you."

It wasn't clear why he moved out after living many months in the hotel, but he connected his departure with bringing legal charges against a fellow tenant. From the hotel, he stayed with a friend for a while, then lived on the streets and at a drop-in center. At about the same time he moved out of the hotel, he quit attending his outpatient clinic and so quit accepting injections of long-acting antipsychotic medication.

Mr. GG. saw no need to attend the clinic. He said its groups were redundant, the same thing over and over. And he saw no need for medication. "It absolutely no way helps me," he said, "I'm an artist. I don't need meds." Besides, he believed it caused him side effects: build-up of fatty tissue on his legs, lethargy, tiredness, and unsteady walking. "Being lethargic is very dangerous when you are on the streets," he said.

When told he would have to take medication in the alternatives to incarceration outpatient program he said he would take it without a problem.

12.2.3 Comment

In an alternatives to incarceration program, Mr. GG. would agree to accept psychiatric treatment, supervised housing, and other services in order to avoid incarceration. Someone would be checking to be sure he took medication. This was a coercive arrangement; he had to do what was expected or go to jail. But less-coercive discharge plans did not stop him from quitting medication and getting arrested for crimes driven by resurgent symptoms of his illness. More coercion and more supervision might prevent more arrests for assault.

12.3 CASE HH: LIVING ON THE STREETS LIKE A DOG

12.3.1 Case

Mr. HH. was close to age 60 when he was arrested for a serious crime and sent to jail. After he was found not fit to stand trial, he was transferred to a state hospital for restoration of fitness.

Interview

On admission interview, Mr. HH. appeared old and worn beyond his years, with oral-buccal movements typical of tardive dyskinesia (TD). All his replies were relevant and not suspicious, but no more than a word or two and offered without expression. He said he had no hallucinations and described his mood as happy.

Course of treatment

Due to his clear and recent history of abuse of substances that could induce psychotic and mood symptoms, Mr. HH.'s diagnosis was not certain. Weeks would pass before the hundreds of pages of his medical records could be collected and reviewed. In the meantime, to clarify his diagnosis and minimize his risk of long-term TD, his doctor stopped the long-acting intramuscular antipsychotic medication he had been accepting while incarcerated and monitored him closely to detect any change.

Therapists who spoke with him and saw him in groups were impressed by his inability to read or write and his simple thinking, so a psychologist administered an IQ test. Mr. HH. told the psychologist that, as a child, he had been in special education classes for learning problems. While doing his best, he scored in a very low range, with a Full Scale IQ score of less than 60.

In subsequent interviews, as in his first, he was placid, unexpressive, and rarely spontaneous. He never voiced delusions and answered questions directly and very briefly. More than once he said he only heard voices when he used illicit drugs, but sometimes he said he did hear voices without using drugs, but they didn't bother him. He attended some therapeutic groups but made no contributions to the discussions, watched television, and played cards with other patients.

With some time and effort, his psychiatrist was able to piece together his history.

History

Mr. HH. was first admitted to a state psychiatric hospital in his early 20s, but his first hospitalization for psychiatric illness, his first arrest, and the start of his excessive drinking all occurred when he was a teenager. He was first admitted after his parents complained he was confused and did not sleep. They believed his main problem was drinking but also reported that he rarely followed-up with scheduled outpatient appointments or took prescribed medication. Psychiatrists started antipsychotic medication because he was paranoid, illogical, and concrete in his thinking.

Mr. HH. disagreed with their assessment. He said, "There's nothing wrong with me. I want discharge. . . . I am leaving this place right now. I don't like being locked up. I will go on the street and take care of my business." After a few months, he was discharged to his parents' home with a community mental health clinic appointment.

Many, many community and state psychiatric hospitalizations ensued. His attitude toward treatment, both outpatient and inpatient, did not change. Mental health professionals struggled to engage him in treatment or at least pin him down and give him supervision. They offered substance abuse treatment. They tried placement in a supervised residence, an intensive case manager (ICM), and assisted outpatient treatment (AOT). Despite their efforts, over more than 30 years, he was arrested numerous times, mostly for drug-related crimes, but also for property crimes and occasionally for assault. His heavy drinking continued, but he also branched out into use of multiple other illicit substances. As psychiatric professionals struggled, so did his family.

Ten years after his first state psychiatric admission, Mr. HH.'s parents complained that he had assaulted his father and threatened to kill all his family. He also talked to himself, didn't sleep regularly, and lived on the streets. By this time, he was described as a chronic abuser of crack cocaine, alcohol, and marijuana. His parents initiated his admission to a community hospital, where he was treated for several months.

By his mid-30s, he had acquired an ICM to monitor and guide his outpatient care. Nevertheless, his parents petitioned to have him admitted to a hospital because he was not bathing, not sleeping, talking to himself, and wandering the streets aimlessly. In a family meeting at a state hospital, his parents told him he could not come home. Mr. HH. did not accept what he heard, but insisted his mother and father really wanted him home and spent his free time pleading with them over the telephone. Over the course of a lengthy stay, his treatment team managed to find a residence willing to accept Mr. HH. Within 2 days of discharge, he walked out of the residence and back into his family's home.

In his 40s, he had more psychiatric admissions, at least one instigated by his parents, one because he did not follow his AOT order, and one because he was found not fit to stand trial on charges of assault. He walked into emergency rooms (ERs) many times and asked for substance abuse or psychiatric services, though ER staff concluded he was really looking for a warm, safe place to sleep and eat. On several occasions, he was taken to ERs after his parents called emergency services. By this time he had an AOT order with an associated ICM.

For a few years, starting in his late 40s, he lived in a residence, at least sometimes. His pattern was to binge on alcohol and illicit drugs, become irritable and sometimes combative, then sleep it off, sober up, and take his medication until the next binge. At times he was brought to an ER by residence staff after he had disappeared for a few days and returned to the residence intoxicated. Other times he walked in on his own asking for medication or a place to stay.

During one hospitalization, inpatient staff succeeded in transferring him to an inpatient substance abuse program. During another, clinicians gave their best effort, but Mr. HH. failed several phone interviews due to irritability and perceived lack of motivation. He was discharged back to his residence with an ACT team.

His reliance on ERs grew when, after a longer than usual incarceration, he did not return to the residence. It redoubled after his mother's death and his father's move to a nursing home. At least once a week he appeared in an ER, often the same one. At times he would walk into an ER complaining of hallucinations telling him to kill himself, but suddenly change his story and just ask for food. "I'll be leaving after I eat," he said. One night he said, "I have nowhere else to sleep. I can't be living in the street like a dog." He told staff he would rather stay in a hospital than a shelter because "they can't mind their own goddamn business in a shelter."

Often he presented with medical problems such as respiratory infections, lice infestation, or skin and wound infections, but he never continued treatment outside the ER. During a cold winter month he appeared in an ER with gangrene due to frostbite in a number of his toes. After his foot was treated, he was discharged with a clinic appointment. Mr. HH. returned to the ER each day for a week for treatment of gangrene.

He often requested but was rarely granted hospital admission. Some psychiatrists believed that he was not psychotic but had behavior problems. Many concluded that he was able to care for himself to a reasonable degree and discharged him from the ER.

Occasionally he was hospitalized, but his ER visits were no less frequent. On one occasion he arrived at an ER thinner than usual, having an animated conversation with someone no one else heard. After he was admitted and restarted on medication, he settled down, but, as discharge neared, he asked for substance abuse rehabilitation but later changed his mind. Mr. HH. was sent back to where he came from. He was admitted again after he arrived at an ER dirty and smelly, disoriented, and mumbling to himself. With medication and time away from alcohol and illicit drugs, his behavior improved and he was discharged to a shelter. Less than a week after he was discharged, he was admitted to another hospital.

After about a year in jail, he walked into an ER complaining of hallucinations telling him to kill himself. He admitted to using multiple illicit substances that could cause hallucinations, and, 3 days after he was admitted, he was discharged. Within a few days he was readmitted to the same hospital, treated for about a month, and discharged. Then, a few days later, he was arrested for a serious crime and incarcerated.

Course of treatment continued

Within weeks after his long-acting injectable antipsychotic was stopped, ward attendants complained he was more irritable and acting strangely. Mr. HH. complained of poor sleep and voices laughing at him, which made him angry. He said that, for a few weeks, his mood had been shaky and depressed. He asked for medication, and his psychiatrist immediately prescribed it.

While he never tried to assault anyone, complaints about him continued. A social worker said he was more abrupt and irritable. Other ward staff reported that he raised his voice, banged on a table, and did not shower. In an interview with his psychiatrist, he was smelly and restless, abrupt and irritable. He said voices had been yelling and laughing at him for a few weeks; they made him angry and violent.

Several weeks after restarting antipsychotic medication, he was no longer smelly and irritable. He said his mood was happy and reported that his most recent hallucinations, voices shouting at him, had occurred a few days earlier. He was found fit to stand trial and discharged to prison with a diagnosis of schizophrenia and intellectual disability.

12.3.2 Comment

Mr. HH. was a man at risk for violence who was also unable to care for himself. Over many years, efforts to manage his risk in the community, such as ICMs,

AOT, and a supervised residence, could not keep him off the streets and out of jail for long. However, he fared better with these services than without them.

After an incarceration, he lost supervision, housing, and connection to clinicians who knew him well and so lost continuity of care. Instead, he relied on ER services. Clinicians who saw him in ERs and in community hospitals did not replace the services he had earlier. Mr. HH.'s diagnosis was clouded by substance abuse and incomplete due to the unavailability of his extensive treatment records, so some psychiatrists failed to appreciate that he had schizophrenia. Some did not seem to understand his limitations or saw his problems as "behavioral."

This case is an example of the problem of disentangling "mad" from "bad." To categorize Mr. HH. as only "bad" would imply that his behavior should be addressed by the criminal justice system, not by psychiatric care and treatment. Both are a means to address dangerous behavior. Both provide containment.

When psychiatrists believed he was a suitable candidate for psychiatric treatment and admitted him to hospital, he was discharged after short stays. His symptoms mostly cleared, he was impatient for discharge, and a wait for a state hospital transfer could be lengthy. Psychiatrists may have felt a legal obligation to release him because they believed he was not imminently dangerous. But Mr. HH. could have been retained or referred to a state hospital because he was unable to care for himself. His long history demonstrated that he was unable to live safely in the community even with an array of supports.

12.4 ARREST AND INCARCERATION

12.4.1 Rates of arrest

Individuals with serious psychiatric illness treated in a public mental health system have high rates of criminal justice involvement (Swanson et al., 2013), arrest (Cuellar et al., 2007; Fisher et al., 2006), and incarceration (Cox et al., 2001; Hawthorne et al., 2012). This was determined by case match studies, which identify individuals with serious psychiatric illness treated in a public mental health system and then search for them in criminal justice records. Rates are hard to compare due to differences in study methods and may change with time and local practices, such as diversion or crisis intervention teams. Fisher's (2006) study demonstrated that, as in the general population, a small number of individuals accounted for a disproportionate number of arrests. Five percent of arrestees accounted for 17% of all arrests.

In these studies, arrests in people treated in the public psychiatry system were usually for minor crimes and rarely resulted in severe criminal sanctions (Cox et al., 2007; Cuellar et al., 2007; Fisher et al., 2006; Swanson et al., 2013). Cuellar's group found that half of arrests resulted in case dismissed or suspended with no further action, while 47% resulted in conviction with sentence, fine, probation, or restitution. Cox's group found that fewer than 3.5% of those who spent at least one night in jail were also incarcerated in prison. Of arrests of adults treated in the public psychiatric system in Connecticut (Swanson et al., 2013), close to half (43%) were for minor crimes such as trespass, breach of peace, and driving while intoxicated (DWI). Twenty-one percent were for property crimes, 15% for drug crimes, and 10% for violent offenses.

In Massachusetts, investigators (Fisher et al., 2011) compared rates of arrest among adults treated in the state public psychiatric system to rates in a comparable subset of the general population. The odds of being arrested at least once for any crime were significantly greater for the mentally ill group (odds ratio [OR], 1.62). Investigators also compared rates of arrest for categories of charges. The risk of arrest was greater for the mentally ill group for all categories of charges, but the odds ratios were larger for less-serious offenses such as crimes against public decency (such as prostitution), misdemeanor crimes against property and against persons, and crimes against public order. An exception was the more serious offense, assault and battery on a police officer, which was almost six times more likely in the mentally ill group.

In a different approach (Compton et al., 2023), a review of all New York state arrests, excluding traffic and vehicular charges from 2010 to 2013, compared arrests of people with serious mental illness (SMI) to arrests of people without. Misdemeanors such as petit larceny, third-degree assault, and making graffiti were substantially more common in arrests of people with SMI. The most common was for trespass, comprising 2.5% of arrests of people with SMI versus 1.7% of arrests of people without SMI. Larceny-theft (e.g., shoplifting) was 20% more common in arrests of SMI individuals. Violent crimes were a smaller percentage of the total of crimes for which people with SMI were arrested, 7.3% vs. 7.6% for people without SMI.

12.4.2 Results of arrest

Many of the patients in this casebook arrived at state hospitals via an arrest and a finding of not fit to stand trial. Often their charges were misdemeanors and so were dropped. Readers should not assume that this is the typical experience for people with SMI who are arrested. In 2016, in New York state there were 328,058 misdemeanor arrests, but only 710 cases were dropped due to incompetence to stand trial (Hall et al., 2019).

There is evidence that defendants with SMI are more likely to be sentenced to jail time for a misdemeanor offense than defendants without. (Alternate dispositions include diversion to treatment, release on bail, or dismissal of charges.) Investigators (Hall et al., 2019) matched records of about 600,000 people arrested in New York state from 2010 through 2013 to public mental health records. They found that treatment for SMI in the year prior to arrest for a misdemeanor significantly increased odds of a jail sentence (OR, 1.52). Likelihood of a prison sentence after an arrest for a felony was not significantly different for the SMI and control groups, but the odds of a prison sentence for a violent crime were 46% greater for the SMI group. The results were independent of the individual's criminal history.

12.4.3 Rates of SMI in jails

Studies of the population of jails and prisons for adults consistently find elevated rates of mental illness. Jails are facilities operated by local entities—usually counties or cities—that hold both inmates who are awaiting trial and those who have been convicted and are either awaiting sentencing or serving a sentence of less than 1 year. Jails are short-term, rapid-turnover facilities. Prisons are longer-term facilities run by states or the federal government that typically hold felons and persons with sentences of more than a year (Bureau of Justice Statistics, n.d.).

Two groups used rigorous methods of detection and definition to estimate the proportion of jail populations with a serious mental disorder. Teplin and colleagues (1994) used a narrow definition of mental illness in a study of 728 randomly selected male detainees in a Chicago jail. Extensively trained clinical psychologists conducted interviews during jail intake using a widely accepted diagnostic structured interview to determine rates of current (within 2 weeks of interview) and lifetime psychiatric disorders. Only 5% of inmates refused interview. SMI was defined as one of schizophrenia, mania, or major depressive disorder. Of the jail population at the time, 56% were charged with misdemeanors and 44% with felonies. All were men.

Of the jail population, 48% met criteria for current antisocial personality disorder (ASPD), 29% had a current substance use disorder, and 6% met criteria for current serious mental disorder. Percentages for lifetime disorders were higher: 49% for ASPD, 61% for substance use disorder, and 9% for SMI.

Detainees with any current SMI had significantly higher rates of comorbid drug and alcohol use disorders than did detainees without current SMI, but there was no similar difference for ASPD (Abram & Teplin, 1991). Of the lifetime SMI group, almost all (94%) had lifetime drug or alcohol disorders or ASPD. Most of the lifetime SMI group (69%) had lifetime ASPD, but only the SMI individuals charged with felonies were more likely to have ASPD than the non-ill group. Also, SMI men were significantly more likely to report alcohol and drug use at the time of arrest compared to the non-ill group.

Teplin (1990) then compared prevalence in a Chicago jail to prevalence in a sample of the general population that was selected for age, gender, and race to be comparable to the jail population. Rates in the general US population were estimated by the Epidemiologic Catchment Area (ECA) Study (Regier et al., 1988), which used the same diagnostic tool used in the jail study. Current and lifetime prevalence rates for each of major depressive disorder, mania, and schizophrenia were all significantly higher in jail than in the general population. Rates for any of the three current disorders was 6.36% in jail and 1.84% in the ECA study, and lifetime rates were 9.48% in jail and 4.41% in the ECA Study.

Steadman and colleagues (2009) used careful methods of detection but defined mental illness more broadly. Between 2002 and 2006, the group selected 822 recently incarcerated men and women at five jails in Northeastern US states. Jail detainees were administered a well-accepted structured diagnostic interview by thoroughly trained interviewers. However, interviewers did not measure functional impairment, thus possibly overestimating rates. SMI was defined as one of six psychotic disorders and five affective disorders. These included schizophrenia, bipolar 1 disorder, and major depressive disorder. Across jails, the rate of past month SMI for male inmates was 14.5% and for female inmates 31.0%. Adding PTSD to the criteria for SMI led to rates of 17% for men and 34% for women.

12.4.4 Rates of SMI in prisons

Reported estimates of the prevalence of mental illness in prisons vary widely. In a 2014 review of 28 studies published between 1989 and 2013 of people incarcerated in state prisons (Prins, 2014), estimates for current major depressive disorder ranged from 9% to 29%, for bipolar disorder from 5.5% to 16.1%, and for schizophrenia from 2% to 6.5%. Rates for substance abuse and personality disorders were not reported.

A later review of health records for all 8,574 prison inmates in Iowa collected data on current and past mental illness as diagnosed by prison clinicians using both the International Classification of Disease (ICD-9) and the *Diagnostic and Statistical Manual of Mental Disorders* (DSM-IV) codes (Al-Rouson, 2017). Ninety-one percent of inmates were men. Eighteen percent had a diagnosis of major depressive disorder, 12% of schizophrenia or a psychotic disorder, and 7.5% bipolar disorder. The majority of the conditions were current, not resolved. Having one of these disorders increased the odds of having a substance abuse disorder, from 4 times for bipolar disorder to 2.5 times for schizophrenia. As in jail populations, rates of personality disorder, at 11%, and substance use disorder, at 26%, were high. Women had higher odds of having both a mental illness and substance use disorder.

REFERENCES

Abram, K. M., & Teplin, L. A. (1991). Co-occurring disorders among mentally ill jail detainees. *American Psychologist* 46(10):1036–1045.

Al-Rouson, T., Rubenstein, L., Sieleni, B., Deol, H., & Wallace, R. B. (2017). Inside the nation's largest mental health institution: A prevalence study in a state prison system. *BMC Public Health* 17:342.

Bureau of Justice Statistics (n.d.). Frequently asked questions. What is the difference between jails and prisons? Accessed on October 21, 2025, from: https://bjs.ojp.gov/frequently-asked-questions?page=1#34-0

Compton, M. T., Zern, A., Pope, L. G., Gesser, N., Stagoff-Belfort, A., de Bibiana, J.T., . . . & Smith, T. E. (2023). Misdemeanor charges among individuals with serious mental illness: A statewide analysis of more than two million arrests. *Psychiatric Services* 74(1):31–37.

Cox, J. F., Morschauser, P. C., Banks, S., & Stone, J. L. (2001). A five-year population study of persons involved in the mental health and local correctional systems. *Journal of Behavioral Health Services & Research* 28(2):177–187.

Cuellar, A. E., Snowden, L. M., & Ewing, T. (2007). Criminal records of persons served in the public mental health system. *Psychiatric Services* 58(1):114–120.

Fisher, W. H., Roy-Bujnowski, K. M., Grudzinkas, A. J., Clayfield, J. C., Banks, S. M., & Wolf, N. (2006). Patterns and prevalence of arrests in a statewide cohort of mental health care consumers. *Psychiatric Services* 57(11):1623–1628.

Fisher, W. H., Roy-Bujnowski, K. M., Grudzinkas, A. J., Wolf, N., Crockett, E., & Banks, S. (2011). Risk of arrest among public mental health services recipients and the general public. *Psychiatric Services* 62:67–72.

Hall, D., Lee, L.-W., Manseau, M. W., Pope, L., Watson, A. C., & Compton, M. T. (2019). Major mental illness as a risk factor for incarceration. *Psychiatric Services* 70(12):1088–1093.

Hawthorne, W. B., Folsom, D. P., Sommerfeld, D. H., Lanouette, N.M, Lewis, M. Aarons, G.A., . . . & Jeste, D. V. (2012). Incarceration among adults who are in the public mental health system: Rates, risk factors, and short-term outcomes. *Psychiatric Services* 63(1):26–32.

Prins, S. J. (2014). The prevalence of mental illness in U. S. state prisons: A systematic review. *Psychiatric Services* 65(7):862–872.

Regier, D. A., Boyd, J. H., Burke, J. D., Rae, D. S., Myers, J. K., Kramer, M., . . . & Locke, B. Z. (1988). One-month prevalence of mental disorders in the United States. *Archives of General Psychiatry* 45:977–986.

Steadman, H. J., Osher, F. C., Robbins, P. C., Case, B., & Samuels, S. (2009). Prevalence of serious mental illness among jail inmates. *Psychiatric Services* 60(6):761–765.

Swanson, J. W., Frisman, L. K., Robertson, A. G., Lin, H.-,J., Trestman, R. L., Shelton, D. A., . . . & Swartz, M. S. (2013). Costs of criminal justice involvement among persons with serious mental illness in Connecticut. *Psychiatric Services* 64(7):630–637.

Teplin, L. A. (1990). The prevalence of severe mental disorder among male urban jail detainees: Comparison with the Epidemiologic Catchment Area Program. *American Journal of Public Health* 80(6): 663–669.

Teplin, L. A. (1994). Psychiatric and substance abuse disorders among male urban jail detainees. *American Journal of Public Health* 84(2):290–293.

12.5 CASE II: MAD OR BAD?

12.5.1 Case

Mr. II. was a young man admitted to a state psychiatric hospital from Hospital C., a general community hospital.

Interview

On admission, his psychiatrist found a large, muscular man who was cooperative as he voiced coherent but frightening paranoid ideas. He said he came to the hospital because men were following him; he could hear their voices, and, if he caught them, he would kill them. For now, they had disappeared, but they were waiting for him to come out onto the streets again so they could torture him. He was stressed out, he said. But, in the same interview, he described his mood as happy and volunteered that he was glad to be in a state hospital where he hoped to obtain Social Security (Supplemental Security Income [SSI]) benefits.

By his account, Mr. II.'s life was dominated first by fights and illicit drugs, and later by psychosis and incarceration. He recalled punching another young boy because the child stepped on his new white sneakers. His first use of street drugs was in his early teens, shortly before he quit school to turn his full attention to work as an illicit drug salesman, the only job he ever held. Within two or three years he began using his life-long, everyday drug of choice, intravenous heroin. A first psychiatric hospitalization soon followed because, as he explained, he could not control himself and there was all kinds of stuff going through his mind driving him crazy.

Mr. II. had lived most of his life behind bars, with a first arrest before age 20 for a violent crime. He said everything comes out worse in jail or prison, including voices. Because of the pressure he got into many fights and often cut his wrists.

History from Hospital C. records

Mr. II. took himself to the emergency room of Hospital C. complaining that agents of the CIA and FBI were following him and had caused him to hear voices by implanting a receiver in his head. He admitted to using heroin, methadone, and alcohol on the day of admission. After admission, he would switch rapidly from angry to silly. He frequently spoke of hallucinations prompting him to hit staff members, and he had carried out such assaults. Initially he was treated with haloperidol, but soon psychiatrists started clozapine. But Mr. II. complained of bowel problems and accused his doctor of trying to poison him, so the doctor stopped clozapine.

Course of treatment

Within a few days of his arrival on the state hospital ward Mr. II. demanded discharge, claiming most of the voices were gone and the others he could deal with. The plan he offered was to live with his mother, obtain SSI benefits, and attend a clinic close to his home. A social worker called his mother and learned that, indeed, she wanted him home to live with her. A bridger visited and found that this plan might work; his mother was caring and willing to have him return, and her home seemed clean and safe.

Meanwhile, Mr. II. refused to attend all therapeutic groups. He offered different explanations. First, he said that he was sleepy, then that he got paranoid in small rooms where patients sit close together. Later, he said he felt fine, but still refused. Rather than attend groups Mr. II. spent his time talking on the phone as well as chatting and joking around amiably with ward staff. At other times, he resisted and defied staff rather than get out of bed on time and in other ways comply with daily ward routine; then he complained that other patients got preferential treatment.

A few weeks into his stay he threw and destroyed a television, later explaining he was angry because he was being poisoned. The next week he accused his social worker of stealing his money and threatened to hurt her if she did not stop. Although he still pressed to leave the hospital within a week or so, he didn't.

History from the following 3 years

Mr. II. was not discharged to his mother's home because she died; instead he moved to the hospital's on-grounds residence and to a state outpatient clinic. In the clinic, he hit a security guard who caught him smoking indoors. The guard pressed criminal charges. Mr. II.'s clinic psychiatrist encouraged the guard to do so, arguing that his patient's behavior was deliberate, premeditated, and calculated.

After arrest for misdemeanor assault and a determination that he was not fit to stand trial, Mr. II. was back in a state hospital, his charges dropped. Again, he destroyed property and threatened to hurt other people, but his treatment team managed to engage him in treatment. Progress came with medication treatment over objection and daily supportive therapy with a male psychologist and with male ward attendants. He attended groups for anger management and for substance abusers. After about a year, with olanzapine and haloperidol decanoate, his auditory hallucinations, paranoid ideas, and dangerous behavior resolved. After a social worker helped him resume a relationship with a family member, he was discharged to his home, to be followed by an assertive community treatment (ACT) team and his probation officer.

Less than a year later he was arrested again, this time for an assault in a convenience store where he was accused of trying to steal a can of beer. Charges were dropped again, and he was transferred from jail to a state hospital. On admission, he declared he was the president of the United States and complained he was harassed by agents of the FBI and CIA. Early in his stay he happened to encounter and recognize another patient whom he believed had cheated him years earlier, and he ran up to attack him. Attendants struggled to restrain him and succeeded. Later, in therapeutic groups, he talked to himself or slept or, when he joined in, claimed the US president wanted to hurt him and his family. He told a nurse that his internal organs were moving in his body.

Because he consistently refused medication, his psychiatrist sought and obtained treatment over objection, to which Mr. II responded. He said that medication kept him out of trouble, but acknowledged that he slacked off at times. Mr. II. was discharged again, but was soon rearrested.

12.5.2 Comment

At his first state hospital admission, Mr. II.'s diagnosis was uncertain. Was it antisocial personality disorder, or schizophrenia? Later, he could be seen as suffering from both. His dangerousness was never in question. With much commitment and effort, clinicians in a state hospital were able to successfully treat his illness and contain him, but, even with a parole officer and an ACT team, he was soon rearrested for a violent crime. Jail provided containment but not the quality of treatment he could get in a hospital.

12.5.3 Antisocial behavior and schizophrenia

At his first admission it was easy to minimize or discount this patient's schizophrenic illness and focus instead on his flagrant antisocial traits. One reason was his lack of negative symptoms and disorganized thinking. That he sought admission for distressing hallucinations and, days later, denied that they were a concern was puzzling. A clinician could suspect he was motivated by a wish to obtain federal entitlements. Geller (1980) wrote of patients who use their psychosis to serve practical needs, as, for example, an inpatient whose symptoms remitted on the day his benefit check arrived.

Antisocial behavior, such as assaults on clinicians, often elicits anger and attempts to retaliate, which can lead to viewing the patient as only or primarily antisocial (Travin & Potter, 1982). When an evaluation takes place in jail or prison, clinicians are more likely to interpret patients' pathology as antisocial. However, both antisocial behavior and traits and schizophrenia can coexist. Antisocial behavior can be an effort to adapt to certain environments.

Antisocial personality disorder cannot be diagnosed when antisocial behavior occurs only during the course of schizophrenia or bipolar disorder (American Psychiatric Association, 2022). By his own telling, Mr. II. engaged in antisocial behavior before he developed psychotic symptoms. More history was needed to be certain, but he likely had conduct disorder before 15 years of age.

12.5.4 Prevention of inpatient violence

At different times Mr. II. was treated with clozapine or olanzapine. In the 12-week study of state hospital inpatients with schizophrenia described in Chapter 5.2, clozapine was superior to haloperidol and olanzapine in reducing assaults, and olanzapine was superior to haloperidol (Krakowski et al., 2006). In that study, those patients with a history of conduct disorder, such as Mr. II., had more frequent and serious assaults than those without (Krakowski et al., 2012). In these individuals, the superiority of clozapine and olanzapine in reducing violence was more marked than in those without such a history. In patients with a history of conduct disorder, clozapine was four times more likely than haloperidol to result in decreased levels of violence. In those without a history of conduct disorder it was three times more likely.

There is much evidence that clozapine is effective in decreasing aggressive and violent behavior in people with schizophrenia and some evidence to support its use for such behavior in people with other disorders, including borderline personality disorder, autistic spectrum disorders, posttraumatic stress disorder, bipolar disorder, and learning disability (Frogley et al., 2012).

Inpatient violence can be prevented when patients with increased risk are identified and closely monitored. Acute psychosis is associated with increased risk, so violence is more frequent close to time of admission (Krakowski et al., 1986). Often, assaultiveness associated with acute psychosis declines sharply with hospital treatment, but in some patients it does not. Researchers (Krakowski & Czobor, 1997) identified 75 state hospital patients with varied diagnoses who were assaultive within the first 2 months after admission and followed them for four weeks. In 41 patients, physical assaultiveness was transient (i.e., it decreased rapidly), while in 34 it was persistent. At the end of 4 weeks, transiently violent patients had better response to treatment than did persistently violent patients. The latter group had significantly higher levels of residual hostility and paranoia.

Patients who have been repeatedly violent are at increased risk for continued assaults. Patients described in Chapter 2.3, Chapter 3.3, and Chapter 5.1 were intensively monitored and treated on specialized wards for patients who were repeatedly violent. These were small-census wards with low patient-to-attendant ratios and one dedicated, full-time psychiatrist. With fewer patients, ward staff were able to devote more attention to each patient and intervene if a physical confrontation seemed imminent. Enhanced monitoring and treatment of patients who have been assaultive can have a significant impact on rates of inpatient violence because investigations have found that a small number of patients are responsible for a disproportionate percentage of aggressive behavior (Barlow et al., 2000; Cooper et al., 1983).

Monitoring can be effective when staff identify patient behaviors that predict assault. They are indeed able to do so, contrary to the view that such incidents are unpredictable, "out of the blue" and due to patients acting on delusions or hallucinations (Cooper et al., 1983). A study using video cameras installed in the dayroom of a state hospital intensive treatment unit for violent patients was able to detect antecedent behaviors in assailant and victim that were specific to assaults (Crowner et al., 2005). In 55 physical assaults between 59 patients, threatening and intrusive behaviors occurred in the 5 minutes preceding 60% of assaults and 10% of control periods. Threatening behaviors were fist shaking, yelling, arguing, and non-forceful pushing. Intrusive behaviors were following, touching, or getting physically close. Eighty percent of patients were diagnosed with schizophrenia or bipolar disorder.

The study suggests that crowding—on wards, in elevators, in dining halls—can precipitate assaults via intrusions on patients' personal space.

REFERENCES

American Psychiatric Association. (2022). *Diagnostic and Statistical Manual of Mental Disorders* (5th ed., TR). Arlington, VA: American Psychiatric Publishing, p. 748.

Barlow, K., Grenyer, B., & Ilkiw-Lavalle, O. (2000) Prevalence and precipitants of aggression in psychiatric inpatient units. *Australia and New Zealand Journal of Psychiatry* 34(6):967–74.

Cooper, S. J., Browne, F. W., McLean, K. J., & King, D.J. (1983). Aggressive behavior in a psychiatric observation ward. *Acta Psychiatrica Scandanavica* 68:386–393.

Crowner, M.L., Peric, G., Stepcic, F., & Lee, Y. (2005). Assailant and victim behaviors immediately preceding assault. *Psychiatric Quarterly* 76(3):243–255.

Frogley, C., Taylor, D., Dickens, G., & Picchioni, M. (2012). A systematic review of the evidence of clozapine's anti-aggressive effects. *International Journal of Neuropsychopharmacology* 15(9):1351–1371.

Geller, M. P. (1980). Sociopathic adaptations in psychotic patients. *Hospital and Community Psychiatry* 31:108–112.

Krakowski, M., & Czobor, P. (1997). Violence in psychiatric patients: The role of psychosis, frontal lobe impairment, and ward turmoil. *Comprehensive Psychiatry* 38(4):230–236.

Krakowski, M., Tural, U., & Czobor, P. (2012). The importance of conduct disorder in the treatment of violence in schizophrenia: Efficacy of clozapine compared with olanzapine and haloperidol. *American Journal of Psychiatry* 178(3):266–274.

Krakowski, M., Volavka, J., & Brizer, D. (1986) Psychopathology and violence: A review of literature. *Comprehensive Psychiatry* 27(2):131–148.

Krakowski, M. I., Czovor, P., Citrome, L., Bark, N., & Cooper, T. B. (2006). Atypical antipsychotic agents in the treatment of violent patients with schizophrenia and schizoaffective disorder. *Archives of General Psychiatry* 63:622–629.

Travis, S., & Potter, B. (1982). Mad or bad? Some clinical considerations in the misdiagnosis of schizophrenia as antisocial personality disorder. *American Journal of Psychiatry* 139(10):1335–1338.

13

DISCHARGE DECISIONS NEAR THE END OF LIFE

This chapter is about clinicians' relationships with patients who have no family to care for or make decisions for them. One case illustrates a choice between paternalism and autonomy. Another case is a story of the potential value of asylum.

13.1 CASE JJ: EVERYBODY GETS OLD AND SICK

13.1.1 Case

Mr. JJ. was a state hospital patient in his late 60s when he met with Mr. P., a social worker, and Dr. D., a psychiatrist, to discuss a plan to discharge him to a nursing home.

Interview

Mr. JJ. was wheeled in to meet Mr. P. and Dr. D. His feet were swaddled in thick, pure white athletic socks and hoisted up on the footrests of his chair. His feet didn't make a move, not even a twitch, throughout his interview. His right arm rested limp in his lap. His mouth had trouble forming words and saliva streamed past his lips. The doctor had to lean in to hear. The social worker gave him a tissue to wipe his mouth, which he did, periodically.

Mr. P.: How are you feeling?
Mr. JJ.: All right.
Mr. P.: How are you being treated?
Mr. JJ.: All right.
Mr. P.: What do you think about moving to a nursing home?
Mr. JJ.: Do I have to go?

He was plaintive, not angry, maybe resigned. He just wanted to go home, to get out of his wheelchair, go home and be himself. He laughed as he recalled living at his former address with the rats.

Dr. D.: You could get stronger in a nursing home with physical therapy. We heard you had a stroke.

Mr. JJ.: It's only that my legs went numb. I could get stronger by going home. I lived for years in my own apartment. You could get dependent on those homes. It takes the life out of you.

Mr. P. acknowledged that everybody wants to be independent. He told Mr. JJ. that he could get stronger there and then go home, that he could not take care of himself, that nursing homes were nice places.

Mr. JJ. did not believe it.

Mr. JJ.: I'll get forgotten there. Those workers, they don't care. And doctors, doctors can't show too much love. You're a nice person. You wouldn't lie to me.

Mr. P.: No, I wouldn't lie. I can tell you, it was the hardest thing I had to do to put my mother in a nursing home. But she couldn't get around anymore. She needed to be there.

Mr. JJ.: Did she die there?

Mr. P.: She did. But you, you're different. You had a stroke. You could get stronger and leave. Everybody gets old and sick.

Mr. JJ. could name his medications but did not know what they did for him. He shrugged and admitted he took them because he had to. He shrugged again when asked if they helped him.

Dr. D. asked, "Why are you in the hospital?"

"I've got a mental illness," Mr. JJ. admitted, "I get angry. I'm a troublesome guy."

When asked about his remote legal charge, Mr. JJ. said the crime did not happen. Dr. D. suggested that he didn't want to hurt anybody, and he agreed.

Getting back to the nursing home question, Mr. JJ. said, "Whatever happens, happens, and, I'll do what you say. I'll do it if you can't find something better for me. I want to live where I did before and have a social worker visit me, like before. I had it made then. I really don't want to go to that kind of place [a nursing home]. I'd rather face the rats." He stretched out his arms to show how long the rats were, one foot long.

History

Mr. JJ. was admitted to a state psychiatric hospital from jail after he was he was charged with a minor crime and found not fit to stand trial. Psychiatrists who found him not fit wrote that he had delusions and disorganized thinking. His life had been characterized by long and intensive drinking and scarred by a conviction for a serious crime for which he spent several years in prison.

Hospital psychiatrists wrote that, in the time he spent in the hospital, he was genial with staff he knew well, respectful, and cooperative. He did not mingle with other patients, but neither did he fight with them. At the same time that he denied he had a mental illness, he accepted treatment with clozapine, and as a result, he was not irritable or preoccupied with delusions. Delusions would only surface when he was questioned about them or in frustrating situations, at which times he claimed he was a general in the US Army. In discussions of his failing physical health or his symptoms of mental illness, he would deny that he had problems or needed to be in the hospital.

A few weeks before his interview he suffered a catastrophic neurologic event, a stroke, which left him incontinent and wheelchair-bound. He had no family able to care for him or to offer advice and emotional support. In the past, his elderly mother had traveled a long distance to visit, but she had not been seen or heard from for years.

13.1.2 Comment

Mr. JJ. listened to his social worker and psychiatrist because he had spent most of his life in institutions and was used to being told what to do by people like them. He was clearly helpless and dependent, but, like almost everybody, he wanted to be independent. He wasn't, had rarely been in the past, and would not be in the future. He had no family to advocate for him or to offer another course.

People who cannot care for themselves have always been with us. Families are expected to care for dependent relatives, but when families cannot, the community takes responsibility. In this case, Mr. P. and Dr. D. were agents of an institution created by the community to fill in for family. They both wanted to comfort and tell the truth, or at least not lie. The truth was that Mr. JJ. could not live in his own apartment but had to leave the state hospital and move to an unfamiliar institution where he knew nobody.

The Revised Declaration of Geneva (Parsa-Parsi, 2017) requires physicians to pledge that, "The health and well-being of my patient will be my first consideration" and "I will respect the autonomy and dignity of my patient." Dr. D. and Mr. P. could not both respect this patient's autonomy and do the best they could for his health and well-being. They had to decide what was best for him.

REFERENCE

Parsa-Parci, R. W. (2017). The revised declaration of Geneva: A modern-day physician's pledge. *Journal of the American Medical Association* 318(20):1971–1972.

13.2 CASE KK: HOW AM I DOING?

13.2.1 Case

Mr. KK. was a patient in his 30s, a long-stay voluntary patient at a state psychiatric hospital who had been admitted after he was found not fit to stand trial and his charges dropped.

Interview

Mr. KK. would traverse the hospital's long, linoleum-paved hospital hallways every morning and afternoon with a bag of mail slung over his shoulder. Entrusted with hospital mail delivery as his paid work program assignment, he had purpose and pride. With a little cash in hand and free access to the hospital snack bar, he could enjoy coffee, soda, sandwiches, burgers, French fries, and chicken sandwiches.

In the course of his rounds, he would greet every hospital employee, every doctor, nurse, therapist, or attendant he had ever met, although he was particularly attached to a few, such as the Protestant chaplain. He was acquainted with nearly all employees and half his fellow patients. When Mr. KK. met a psychiatrist he knew, the doctor offered a smile and a few pleasantries, and then started to hurry down the hallway. The doctor was busy, with many obligations, and wanted to avoid one more demand on his time. But Mr. KK. held on. He articulated his words laboriously, slowly, and imperfectly, pressing for reassurance, repeatedly asking, "How am I doing? Am I doing good? What's going to happen to me?"

History

Mr. KK. had a congenital neurological condition that caused his dysarthria and misled elementary school professionals into believing he had an intellectual disability. His early life was marked by neglect and abandonment. His father left when he was still an infant; his mother was more occupied with drinking and illicit drugs than with the care of her child. Soon after his mother's death, his father sent him to an orphanage, called a "home for children," where he was placed in special classes for the intellectually disabled.

A psychiatric hospitalization before he reached his teens was the first of many, all precipitated by attacks on others and himself. His admitting psychiatrist wrote that, from adolescence, he had affective instability with recurrent outbursts of rage, often brought on by interpersonal rejection.

Hospital course

Within his first several months at the hospital there were occasions when he attacked people who frustrated him, usually hospital employees. He once threw a chicken leg in a dining room in an argument over food. With considerable time, treatment with an antipsychotic and lithium, and psychotherapy, his angry storms abated and he showed no evidence of hallucinations or other psychotic symptoms.

However, he was diagnosed with a serious chronic medical illness that was, when detected, in an early, asymptomatic stage.

Mr. KK. underwent a set of cognitive tests that showed that he was, after all, not intellectually limited but of average overall intelligence, with above average verbal skills. While he understood the test results, he often felt compelled to remind others and himself that he was not retarded. Again and again, he asked to take the same tests, usually after he suffered a slight or others spoke to him harshly.

He used his verbal skills in individual psychotherapy. Working with a young psychology intern Mr. KK. came to understand that he tried to hurt others to protect himself from anticipated attacks, disrespect, or exploitation. He practiced self-restraint and expressed anger through talking or prayer, but he needed to be told he was doing right. When an employee rebuffed him or another patient stole food from him in the dining room or shoved or mocked him, he came back to the intern or other staff for reassurance that he had managed the situation in the right way. Still convinced that others disdained and exploited him, he tried to make friends anyway. He conjured memories of his dead mother and long-absent father. He imagined telling them about the past few decades of his life and that he was sick. Mr. KK. knew he was in bad health and feared dying in the hospital. He wished his father would appear and take him home.

One year, in the spring, he was stricken with acute physical distress and was transferred to a general hospital for symptomatic relief. On his return, his treatment team began to explore discharge to a nursing home that they hoped would be well-suited to provide the medical and nursing care Mr. KK. needed. Mr. KK. worried the idea over and over, asking again and again if he would be sent to a nursing home, which he believed would be depressing because he would be surrounded by aged and dying people. However, the nursing home did not accept him because his medical condition was not sufficiently disabling.

He returned to delivering mail, to traveling up and down the hospital hallways. Every time he met his social worker, he implored, "Am I going home? I don't want to go to a nursing home." He had physical symptoms, but never complained of weakness. Weakness could lead to loss of his freedom to move off the ward.

By early summer, he was in the infirmary, an isolated area for more intensive nursing and medical care. Every day a member of his treatment team visited. He was bored and restless. He asked, "What's going to happen to me? When can I leave? I want to leave today," he said, "Today. Let me go today." He chanted, "SO-dah, So-dah, bring me a So-dah." He handed over a dollar. Every day a psychologist, psychiatrist, social worker, or recreation therapist delivered one can of his favorite sugary carbonated drink and one straw. He drained the can, wiped his mouth, looked up, and said, "Chicken sandwich."

He was briefly released and returned to his ward, from which he could leave to purchase his own chicken sandwiches. However, within days, his medical condition worsened to the extent that he was too sick to stay. After he returned to the infirmary, his medication regimen was changed due to his medical problems. For the first time in many years, he complained of auditory hallucinations. Evil spirits taunted him; they told him to go to hell. New changes in his medications were futile, and, as a consequence, the evil spirits could not be contained and continued to torment him.

By late summer, his physical health had so deteriorated that he was accepted by and discharged to an inpatient hospice program. Within 2 weeks, he was back. The hospice would not tolerate his behavior and so returned him. Mr. KK. was emaciated, barely able to breathe, able to express only a few words at a time. "Am I dying? Am I dying? Am I dying?" he gasped. He begged for food. He ate applesauce, pasta, ice cream, and cups of juice. He wanted more. Hospital employees brought him cake, soda, a sandwich. He ate it all and begged to return to his ward.

He could not return to his ward but returned to the infirmary. Around midnight later in the month he was found in his bed pulseless and breathless, and pronounced dead. His records were scoured for family contacts, but none was found.

Afterward

A few weeks later, there was a memorial service for Mr. KK. presided over by the Protestant chaplain. A gospel choir made up of patients dressed in purple robes stood facing a seated group of patients and staff members from throughout the hospital. Some patients continued to talk to themselves but followed the service and sang with feeling. The service included music, prayer, and a eulogy. After the eulogy, patients and staff members took turns standing and honoring Mr. KK.

INDEX

For the benefit of digital users, indexed terms that span two pages (e.g., 52–53) may, on occasion, appear on only one of those pages.

www.ingramcontent.com/pod-product-compliance
Ingram Content Group UK Ltd.
Pitfield, Milton Keynes, MK11 3LW, UK
UKHW021842241026
476982UK00014B/97

9 780197 800584